Praise for Michelle Cooper's books

'Absorbing, compelling and unforgettable.' *Kirkus Reviews*, starred review

'Fascinating and thoroughly engrossing.' *Bulletin of the Center for Children's Books*, starred review

'Beautifully observed and fascinating in its political and historical detail.' *2011 NSW Premier's Literary Awards Shortlist*

'This meticulously researched book presents another great work from a stellar voice in historical fiction for young adults.' *2011 Kids' Indie Next List*

'Cooper's engagement of politics and her quick, inventive wit give the book its own captivating originality.' *The Horn Book Magazine*

'A fascinating series that should be in every library.' *Read Plus*

'Historical fiction at its most engaging … highly recommended.' *Magpies*

'Cooper's books are a great example of what YA fiction should be – as challenging and informative as they are entertaining.' *Wordcandy*

Dr Huxley's Bequest

A HISTORY *of* MEDICINE *in* THIRTEEN OBJECTS

Michelle Cooper

FitzOsborne Press

Published by FitzOsborne Press
www.fitzosbornepress.com

First published by FitzOsborne Press in 2017
This edition published in 2018

Text and illustrations © Michelle Cooper 2017

The moral right of the author has been asserted.

All rights reserved. No part of this book may be reproduced, recorded or transmitted (except under statutory exceptions provisions of Australian copyright legislation) without the prior permission of the author.

 A catalogue record for this book is available from the National Library of Australia

ISBN 978-0-6481651-3-2 (paperback)

Also available in ebook editions (ePub and Kindle)

Cover design by Nada Backovic
Hippocrates bust and Vesalius skeleton images from Wellcome Library, London (CC BY 4.0). Opium poppy public domain image from Biodiversity Heritage Library, digitized by Missouri Botanical Garden, Peter H. Raven Library. Bee images from iStockphoto/benoitb.
Internal design by Pickawoowoo Publishing Group / DiZign Pty Ltd
Printed by Lightning Source (US/ UK/ AUS/ EUR)

CONTENTS

Chapter One
Afterwards, Rosy always blamed the turtle ... 1

Chapter Two
'I'm convinced that a controlled disrespect
for authority is essential to a scientist.' 13

Chapter Three
'I have no special talents. I am only
passionately curious.' 31

Chapter Four
'The scientific mind does not so much
provide the right answers as ask the right
questions.' 43

Chapter Five
'The deepest sin against the human mind is
to believe things without evidence.' 61

Chapter Six
'Formerly, when religion was strong and
science weak, men mistook magic for medicine ...' 77

Chapter Seven
'Good science and good art both require
imagination.' 91

Chapter Eight
'Science is nothing but trained and organised
common sense.'   107

Chapter Nine
'Chance favours only the prepared mind.'   129

Chapter Ten
'Science moves, but slowly, slowly ...'   151

Chapter Eleven
'Science is much more than a body of
knowledge. It is a way of thinking.'   163

Chapter Twelve
'... now, when science is strong and religion
weak, men mistake medicine for magic.'   185

Chapter Thirteen
'Cured yesterday of my disease, I died last
night of my physician.'   207

Chapter Fourteen
'What is a weed? A plant whose virtues have
not been discovered.'   219

Chapter Fifteen
'In science, the credit goes to the man who
convinces the world, not to the man to whom
the idea first occurs.'   229

Chapter Sixteen
'It is those who know little, not those who
know much, who so positively assert that
this or that problem will never be solved by
science.'   241

Chapter Seventeen
'Mystics exult in mystery and want it to stay mysterious. Scientists exult in mystery for a different reason: it gives them something to do.'   257

Chapter Eighteen
'We've never had a woman in the laboratory before, and we think you'd be a distracting influence.'   277

Chapter Nineteen
'It is a good morning exercise for a research scientist to discard a pet hypothesis every day before breakfast.'   289

Chapter Twenty
'Did science promise happiness? I don't think so. It promised truth ...'   307

Author's Note   315

Bibliography   319

Index   331

CHAPTER ONE

Afterwards, Rosy always blamed the turtle.

'It wasn't the turtle's fault,' said Jaz, as the two girls sat in the courtyard beside the pond, eating salt-and-vinegar chips.

'You weren't *there*, Jaz. You didn't see his evil expression. He knew exactly what he was doing. None of it would have happened without that turtle.'

The turtle in question raised his head and turned his beady yellow gaze upon them.

'Look,' said Rosy. 'He's doing it again. Malevolent, that's what I call him.'

'How do you know it's a boy?'

'He's got a beard.'

Jaz peered closer. 'I think that's a bit of lettuce stuck to its chin.'

'After all that everyone here's done for him, too,' Rosy went on. 'Feeding him. Cleaning his stupid pond. And how did he repay us? With treachery and disloyalty and, and … dirty tricks! Just imagine the disaster that would have befallen this college if *we* hadn't come to the rescue.'

'Well, considering there wouldn't have *been* a problem if you hadn't –'

'Malicious,' Rosy said quickly. 'That's what he is. Mephistophelean.'

'That is not even a word.'

'It is. It's from Mephistopheles. Remember, that stone demon spitting into the fountain in Science Road?'

'Oh, right,' said Jaz. 'Faust. The quest for knowledge.'

'Exactly,' said Rosy.

The turtle lunged at a passing dragonfly, snapping off its wing and a couple of legs. The unfortunate insect tumbled onto the surface of the pond and the turtle gulped it down, then twisted his wrinkled, serpentine neck in the direction of the girls.

'He does look a bit sinister,' Jaz conceded.

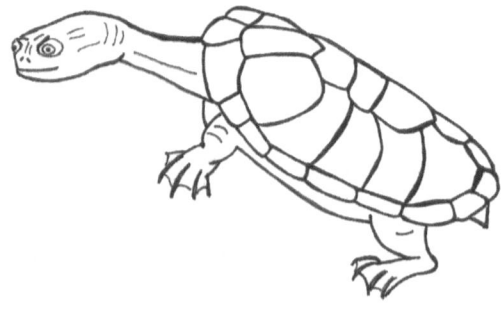

But actually, the whole thing *hadn't* started with the turtle. It had really begun about ten minutes before the turtle made his first fateful appearance, when Rosy's mother – stuffing papers into her satchel, preparing to rush out the door – had asked Rosy to try and keep out of trouble.

The two of them were still in that delicate phase of readjusting to each other after a lengthy separation, so

Chapter One

Rosy didn't snap back. She merely pointed out, very politely, that she was thirteen now and quite capable of looking after herself for a morning without getting into trouble.

'Yes, I'm sure you are,' said Alison, her mum, sounding the exact opposite of sure. 'I just wish that babysitter had turned out to be more ... appropriate. She could have taken you to the pool.'

Honestly! Was there a more insulting word in the universe than 'babysitter', when you were nearly as tall as your mum and had already finished an entire year of high school? Also, Rosy didn't think a pentagram tattoo and an eyebrow ring shaped like a snake swallowing its own tail were all *that* scandalous. It was art, wasn't it? Body art. On the other hand, she really hadn't wanted Mrs Adam's seventeen-year-old niece bossing her around these holidays. Now that Rosy was here in this fascinating old place, she needed to be free to *explore*.

'I don't want to go swimming, Mum,' she said firmly. 'I'm going to walk around and look at all the gargoyles and do some drawings.'

'Well ...' Alison frowned and patted her pockets as the buzzing from her mobile phone grew louder. 'I should be back for lunch, but if you get hungry, go down to the kitchen and make yourself a sandwich. That's next to the refectory –'

'I know. We had dinner there last night, remember?'

'And maybe you can find that other girl, the gardener's daughter? She looks about your age. You probably have lots in common.'

Rosy seriously doubted that. She had seen the girl climbing out of her father's ute that morning and had observed that she:

a) wore nerdy glasses

and

b) carried around a Year Eight Advanced Mathematics workbook.

The probability of Rosy having anything in common with someone who did maths in the summer holidays was approximately zero. Either this girl's father was making her do it, in which case she was a wimp, a suck-up or just pathetic, or else she was doing it for fun, which was plain crazy. But Rosy didn't say any of this to her mother – who, for all Rosy knew, did maths all the time these days, for work *and* fun – and simply stated that a certain person was going to be late for her meeting and also, that her phone was about to vibrate off the window ledge.

'Oh, I wonder how it got there!' said Alison, snatching it up. She'd put it down there herself, three minutes ago, when she was searching for her keys. You'd never guess the woman had two PhDs and had won a university medal for being a genius.

But that was scientists for you, thought Rosy, as her mum dashed off. Brilliant at figuring out the secrets of germs or blood or whatever it was, but not so good at practical, everyday life. Fortunately, Rosy lived most of the time with her dad, who was an artist.

Anyway, now Rosy had an entire morning all to herself and she couldn't wait to start exploring. She wandered down a long corridor lined with panelled

Chapter One

oak doors and emerged into the sudden brightness of the college foyer. The front doors were closed, but light from the stained-glass windows splashed all over the parquet floor, splattering the walls with glorious hues of sapphire and ruby and emerald. There was a wide wooden staircase with elaborately carved banisters, and behind these stairs, an archway that offered an intriguing glimpse of a shadowed stone passageway.

But Rosy decided she would investigate this later. She slid all the way across the foyer (they kept the floors *very* well waxed), past the refectory doors (currently blocked by a cleaner's cart), past a glass-fronted noticeboard and a cabinet full of trophies and sepia photographs, and found herself beside a doorway labelled 'BURSAR'.

She had no idea what BURSAR meant, so she stopped and peeked round the open door. Evidently, BURSAR meant 'very messy office'. There were the usual desks and computers and filing cabinets, as well as a bulky old photocopier, but also – sitting in the middle of the room – a large cardboard carton, out of which had spilled a vast quantity of those fat squashy yellow pellets used to pack fragile items. The pellets appeared almost *alive* – as Rosy watched, a bunch of them rolled, commando-style, under a table and spread out along the wall, as if awaiting further orders.

Ankle-deep in pellets stood three people: a grey-haired woman in capri pants and a cheerful Hawaiian shirt; a scowling younger woman with a helmet of shiny black hair that looked as though it'd been lifted off a Lego figurine; and Nerdy Maths Girl. Rosy might have moved on then, except that Nerdy Maths Girl chose that moment to say, 'Could I have the keys to the Crypt, please?'

Wait, this place had a *crypt*? Awesome! Rosy leaned all the way through the doorway.

'One moment,' said Lego Lady, raising a finger at Nerdy Maths Girl, before turning back to the older woman. 'I specifically told them to deliver this box to the Senior Common Room – I even unlocked the door for them! And whatever possessed you to open it, Lynette? Look at all this, this … this *mess*!' She kicked out at the pellets.

'Don't worry,' said Rosy helpfully. 'They're biodegradable. Totally friendly to the environment.'

The three of them turned to stare at her. Lego Lady's eyes bulged, not in a very friendly way, and Nerdy Maths Girl said hurriedly, '*I* can carry the box up to the Senior Common Room for you. I'll get it out of your way.'

What a suck-up. Rosy tried not to roll her eyes. A crypt would be wasted on that girl. She probably just wanted to do maths in there. Also, anyone with half a brain could see that carton would need more than one person to carry it –

'Would *you* do us a favour and help Jasminder take it upstairs?' said the older woman, sending Rosy a sweet smile. 'It's not very heavy, just an awkward size.'

'Sure,' said Rosy, stepping forward. (Look how obliging she was being! It showed how unfair her mum had been, with all that talk about keeping out of trouble! Plus, Rosy now had an opportunity to explore the Senior Common Room, whatever that was.) 'What's in this box, anyway?' she asked.

Lego Lady snorted. 'It is a collection of artefacts bequeathed to this college by the late Dr Timothy Huxley. As if we didn't *already* have enough old things cluttering up this place.'

'That big glass cabinet in the common room is empty now,' said Lynette, who was trying – without much success – to tape the top flaps of the carton back together while the pellets inside made vigorous escape bids. 'Dr Bennet took all her books out of it when she left last term.'

'Fine,' said Lego Lady, throwing up her hands. 'Girls, put everything on display in there. Apparently, there's a piece of paper in the carton too, explaining what everything is. Pin it up on the noticeboard or stick it in the cabinet, wherever you can find space. Just get this mess out of my office!'

Rosy and the other girl picked up the carton, shuffled through the doorway and headed towards the foyer.

'I'm Rosy, by the way,' said Rosy. 'My mum's going to live here and be a tutor for a semester. She's just come back from three years lecturing at Cambridge University, in England. And you're, um, Jasmin –'

'Jaz.'

'Cool. So, what was that you were saying about a crypt?'

Jaz ignored this. 'The quickest way to the Senior Common Room is through *here*,' she said sternly, as if Rosy had insisted they take some other, utterly mad route – over the Sydney Harbour Bridge, for instance, or via Bondi Beach. Jaz steered them through the stone passageway Rosy had noticed earlier and they came out into a spacious courtyard, paved in worn grey flagstones and furred with moss in the corners. A pond at the far end was surrounded by a rock garden and shaded by a couple of palm trees that rustled in the breeze. Rosy glanced around with interest.

'Watch where you're going,' said Jaz, even though their progress had been perfectly smooth. 'It's up the top of those steps. I'd better go first.'

'Why?'

'Because whoever goes first has to walk backwards,' said Jaz. 'And you're more likely to trip over.'

'How would you know?' said Rosy, starting to feel quite irritated with this girl. '*You're* the one wearing glasses, not me.'

'But *I've* been up here before,' said Jaz and she forestalled further argument by starting up the steps herself. Rosy really *did* roll her eyes this time, but she followed without protest. It was already taking most of her concentration, balancing her end of the carton while trying to hold the top flaps closed with her chin. And although the carton wasn't truly heavy, she wouldn't have minded putting it down for a moment to readjust her grip.

Jaz must have felt the same, because when she reached the landing halfway up, she said, 'You can have a break here, if you want.'

'Oh, how generous of you,' said Rosy with withering sarcasm, although Jaz's expression didn't even flicker.

Chapter One

They lowered the carton onto the landing and Jaz tried to stick down the flaps again.

'Wait, there's something caught underneath,' said Rosy, and she reached into the carton and tugged out a piece of paper – no, two pieces of paper, as flimsy as onion skin and covered in shaky blue writing. 'Hey, look! This must be about the collection, explaining what all these things are.'

'Put those papers back,' ordered Jaz, hands on her hips.

Rosy had never met anyone her own age so incredibly *bossy*. 'I'm having a break,' she said, focusing on trying to decipher the writing. Jaz reached over and Rosy twisted away, holding the papers higher. 'Stop that! You'll make me –'

'Careful of the box!' cried Jaz, and as they both turned to nudge the carton closer to the wall, a sly breeze twitched the papers out of Rosy's fingers. For a few seconds, the papers hovered above the girls' heads, tantalisingly close. Then a fresh gust swept one piece of paper even higher, while the other spiralled down, down, down into the courtyard.

Rosy and Jaz turned identical horrified looks upon each other, then raced off in opposite directions – Jaz up the stairs, where one paper was now dancing along the wide railing, while Rosy hurtled downwards, making wild snatches at the air. She vaulted the last three steps, then almost tripped into the pond, where the paper had come to rest on top of the water.

'Don't you *dare* move,' she muttered, climbing onto the ledge of the pond. She leaned over, stretching out her hand to its limits, nearly, *nearly* ... and there it was. She had it!

But just as she grasped it, a tiny crocodile exploded out of the water and snapped at her fingers.

'Arrgh!' cried Rosy, lurching sideways. The creature responded by clamping its jaws around the paper and trying to drag it underwater. Rosy, clinging to the rock that had saved her from a dunking, now saw that her adversary was actually a turtle with evil little eyes.

'Give that back!' she told the turtle. 'You don't want it – it's not *food*!' She extended one arm, grabbed the edge of the paper and pulled. There was a brief but intense tug of war.

Rosy lost.

'Now look what you've done!' she ranted, holding up the corner she'd managed to save. The turtle smirked and dived back under the water, while Rosy groped about for a stick, hoping to rescue the rest of the paper before the turtle tried to eat it. She'd just managed to retrieve the sodden mass from the bottom of the pond when Jaz rushed up, panting.

'It got away from me!' she wailed. 'It kept floating higher and higher, and then it blew off over the roof and got caught in that big gum tree!' Then she saw what Rosy was trying to spread out on the ground – the wad of paper, now smeared with mud, its words blurred beyond recognition – and all the colour drained from Jaz's face.

Rosy looked at Jaz and then she looked back down at the paper. She remembered her mum telling her to keep out of trouble, and she experienced a horrible sinking sensation. Almost as if she really *had* fallen into the depths of a nasty, murky pond.

CHAPTER TWO

'I'm convinced that a controlled disrespect for authority is essential to a scientist.'
~ Luis W. Alvarez

'Don't worry,' Rosy told Jaz, with more confidence than she felt. 'Look, we've still got this.' From the pocket of her shorts, she retrieved the scrap of paper she'd ripped from the turtle's jaws. They bent their heads over the paper. It said:

1. Ancient Egyp
2. Stone Head of

'Oh, that's really helpful,' said Jaz. 'Really informative!'

'There's no need to panic,' said Rosy. 'Just … take a deep breath, okay? Now … another one. Anyway, there's probably an extra copy of these notes in the box.'

Suddenly reminded of the carton's existence, they whipped their heads round to check on it. It wouldn't have surprised Rosy to see it had tumbled down the stairs and smashed itself to smithereens, the way things were going. But no, there it sat safely on the landing, still dribbling pellets.

'Let's just get it into the common room,' said Jaz, and they carried it very gingerly up the remainder of the stairs, along a balcony and through the doorway.

The Senior Common Room proved to be a large shadowy room fitted out with a lot of leather armchairs and cedar bookcases and threadbare Persian rugs. The girls made their way over and around all this to the sturdy glass-fronted cabinet in the corner. 'Locked,' said Jaz, trying its door.

'Never mind,' said Rosy. 'Let's unpack all the things and put them on the table for now. Turn that lamp on, will you?'

They opened the carton and began lifting out various strange and wonderful objects. There was a translucent yellow-orange blob, like a dollop of honey turned to stone, wrapped in a square of blue velvet.

There was a framed illustration of a skeleton leaning against a tomb – apparently from a very old book, because there was a page number in the top corner and the writing was in Latin. There were also some fragments of old print, in English, but no easier to understand.

There was a creepy porcelain head with a hole in its throat and writing all over its bald scalp. There was a pink cardboard packet labelled 'ASPRO' – which turned out to be empty – and a faded little box stamped 'Dried Smallpox Vaccine NOT FOR INJECTION' – which rattled when Rosy picked it up, although neither of them was brave enough to open it.

Chapter Two

There was another head, this one of pale stone, depicting an old man with a long, curly beard; a small leather case that flipped open to reveal a medallion; a tiny painting of a figure with a gold halo; and a thick, shiny metal spiral the length of Rosy's hand.

At the bottom of the carton sat two identical mahogany boxes, each lined with padded velvet. The first box contained a sealed glass flask, half full of a brownish liquid; the second held a bizarre contraption made of tin, consisting of a tennis-ball-sized sphere with a number of attachments. After stirring around in the pellets littering the base of the carton, Jaz drew out the thirteenth object: a beautiful little turquoise ornament in the shape of an eye.

But there were no more pieces of paper.

'They might have got stuck in the sides of the box,' said Rosy, peeling the cardboard flaps apart. Her worries had retreated as she'd got caught up in the fascinating process of revealing each object, but now they all rushed back with sickening force. There was no sign of any other papers – not under the flaps or wedged in the corners of the carton or folded inside the mahogany boxes. Jaz sifted frantically through the pile of discarded pellets. Nothing. Rosy turned the empty carton upside down and gave it a thump. All that produced was a cloud of yellow dust that made them sneeze.

But then Jaz spotted something.

'What's that?' she said, pointing at the head of the old man. On his neck, almost hidden in the curls of his beard, was a tiny round sticker, with '2' written on it in blue ink.

'That's the number on my scrap of paper!' said Rosy. 'See, it says item two is a stone head of ... well, it must be this old guy, whoever he is. And item one is an ancient Egypt ... thing. Hey, the eye ornament – *that* looks Egyptian!' She snatched it up. 'Oh. Its sticker must have fallen off.'

They examined the other objects, but only the two wooden boxes had retained their numbers, probably because those stickers had been placed inside their lids. The flask was numbered '5' and the tin contraption was '6'.

'All the other stickers must have been rubbed off inside the carton,' said Rosy, and when they searched through the pellets, they did indeed discover a couple of dusty, curled-up, no-longer-attached stickers.

'This is bad,' said Jaz, shaking her head. 'This is really, *really* bad. A valuable collection bequeathed to this college – and we've destroyed the only explanation of it!'

'Well, it wasn't as though it was a very *good* explanation,' said Rosy. 'It was just handwritten notes – and not very detailed notes, either. I mean, how could anyone possibly explain that weird tin thing in a couple of words? They didn't even manage to stick the numbers on properly.'

Jaz dropped her head into her hands and moaned. 'I'm going to be in so much trouble! *I* offered to carry it up here. I was responsible for it. And now –'

Chapter Two

'Actually, *I* was the one who took the notes out of the carton in the first place,' said Rosy. 'So it's more my fault than yours.' Of course, the papers would have been completely safe if Jaz hadn't been so bossy and tried to grab them. But Jaz was looking so distraught that Rosy couldn't help feeling sorry for her. 'Anyway, your dad's the gardener here, right? They know you. So they'll know how careful you usually are and they'll understand this was just a mistake.'

'But he's *not* the gardener!' wailed Jaz. 'He's got a contract to do the landscaping in the front, and he only started yesterday, and it's his first big contract, and if he does well at this and they like him, he might get more work here at the university and we really need the money, but when they find out that I've –'

'Stop!' said Rosy. 'Now, *breathe*. Slowly.' She waited for Jaz to stop hyperventilating. 'Look. We'll go downstairs and tell them what happened and they'll all blame me. They're not going to sack my mum, because she's a really famous scientist and they're lucky to have her here. Mind you, she's going to hit the roof and take away all my pocket money and tell my dad and he'll do that I'm-not-angry-I'm-disappointed thing, but it's fine. Really.'

'But –'

'Oh, come on, let's get it over with. We need to ask for the key to that cabinet, anyway. We can't leave these things sitting around on a table.'

Rosy seized Jaz's arm and dragged her back along the scattered trail of yellow pellets to BURSAR, where Lynette had just finished cleaning up the carpet.

'Everything all right?' the older woman said, setting her dustpan and brush down. 'That box wasn't too heavy for you, was it?'

'No, no, it was fine,' said Rosy, relieved to see Lego Lady wasn't there. 'But, um, we need the key to unlock the cabinet.'

'Oh, of course,' said Lynette, pulling open the drawer of her desk. 'Here you go. Is there enough room inside the cabinet for all the things?'

'Yes, I think so,' said Rosy. 'Er, but there *is* something I need to –'

Lego Lady stalked back into the room at that moment, waving a file. 'Here it is, Lynette, that list of painters. Now we'll be able to get the entire wing painted, not just the part where the roof leaked! Perhaps even new carpet – get some quotes for that as well, will you?'

'Isn't it marvellous?' said Lynette to the girls. 'That nice man who bequeathed us all those old things has left the college one hundred and fifty thousand dollars in his will!'

'Oh,' said Rosy weakly. 'That's ... nice.'

'Yes, it's all set out in this letter from his solicitor. All we have to do in return is provide a secure display space for his lifetime's collection of artefacts.'

Jaz gave an audible gulp.

'Was there ... um, anything *else* enclosed in the letter?' Rosy asked.

'Unfortunately not.' Lego Lady didn't look up from her papers. 'I wish they'd enclosed a cheque. But that's lawyers for you, always have to make things

Chapter Two

complicated. Oh no, they can't give us the money until they've come out and inspected the display and ensured that the terms of his will have been met!'

'They're just doing their job,' said Lynette. 'But imagine – we might even be able to get a new photocopier!'

'Don't get too excited,' said Lego Lady. 'Although maybe now the College Board will consider landscaping the entire grounds. They could get rid of those horrible old shrubs that scrape the side of my car whenever I park round the back.'

'Yes, that would be wonderful,' said Lynette, with a sigh. Then she turned to Rosy. 'But how rude of me, I interrupted you. What were you about to say?'

'Um, I was just going to say that, that …'

Rosy glanced at Jaz, who twisted her hands together and sent Rosy an imploring look.

Rosy took a deep breath and plunged in. 'I was going to say that because the artefacts are so important and valuable, I think they need proper labels, explaining what they all are. But the notes supplied in the carton were … er, not really adequate. Were they, Jaz?'

Jaz shook her head violently.

'They were just very brief handwritten notes,' said Rosy. 'We could hardly read them, could we? So we – Jaz and I – thought we'd like to do proper labels on the computer, printed out so that everyone can read them, with some extra research that explains more about all the … things.'

'Oh, what a good idea!' cried Lynette, turning to Lego Lady. 'Isn't that a good idea?'

'Yes, fine,' said Lego Lady, shuffling through her file. 'Just make sure it's all done by the time that solicitor comes out here. Lynette, what was the name of that electrician, the one who rewired the kitchen?'

'When would that be?' said Rosy. 'When's the solicitor coming out?'

Lego Lady gave her a quizzical look over the top of her papers. 'When we call to arrange it, I expect.'

'How long will it take to get the display all set up, girls?' asked Lynette, reaching for the diary on her desk.

'Maybe a week –' said Rosy.

'Two,' squeaked Jaz.

'A week or two,' Rosy said. 'Probably two.'

'There, I've made a note to call their office,' said Lynette. 'Thanks, girls. Aren't you good to spend your holidays doing this! I can't wait to see what all those things are – Oh, good morning, Ferdinand! How are *you* today?'

A small man brandishing a mop had just marched into the room. 'How am I?' he snapped. 'How *am* I? I come out of the refectory and what do I find? Little bits of yellow foam, all over my clean foyer floor!'

Rosy felt she'd taken responsibility for enough problems that morning. She grabbed Jaz and they fled.

Back in the common room, they collapsed into adjacent armchairs to catch their breath. Rosy still couldn't believe they'd actually gotten away with it.

Chapter Two

Jaz was the first to state the obvious. 'How are we going to make labels for all these things? We don't have the slightest clue what they are!'

'That's totally not true,' Rosy said, because there was something about Jaz that simply *compelled* Rosy to argue with her, even when Jaz was saying exactly what Rosy had been thinking. 'We *do* have some clues. Like, we know what the first one is. It's an ancient Egyptian ... eye thing. And that stone head is probably some really famous guy. Otherwise, why would they have bothered making a sculpture of his head? He looks ancient Greek to me.'

'Or Roman,' said Jaz, because she was so contrary and annoying.

'Or Greek,' Rosy shot back, thinking Jaz could at least show some gratitude to Rosy for getting them out of trouble. Or out of *one* sort of trouble. She was starting to think she might have gotten them into a whole different lot of trouble.

'Where do we even begin our research?' said Jaz, gnawing at her lower lip. 'We need a plan.'

'We need to make a list!' said Rosy, because she'd just bought herself an excellent set of fluorescent glitter pens.

'We need to lock these things inside the cabinet before anything else happens to them,' said Jaz, and Rosy couldn't argue with that. They also agreed to arrange the objects in the cabinet from oldest to most modern.

'I bet that's what the numbers on the stickers mean,' said Rosy. 'The scrap of paper says the ancient Egypt thing is number one and you can't get much older than ancient Egypt, can you?'

'Well, there's the Stone Age,' said Jaz, as she placed the turquoise eye ornament on the very top shelf. 'But are you *sure* this is Egyptian? Maybe it's Aztec or something.'

'Maybe. Except there wasn't anything *else* in that box that looks like it might have come from ancient Egypt.' Rosy leaned in to examine the ornament. 'It's so pretty, isn't it? There's a loop attached, too. I think it used to be part of a necklace.'

'Next comes the stone head,' said Jaz, cradling it in her hands. 'From ancient Rome.'

'Or ancient Greece,' said Rosy. 'Are you certain there's nothing written on it? Hold it up higher so I can check underneath ... Aha! Words from antiquity, carved into the stone by ancient hands!'

'What? What does it say?'

'*Made in China*. No, I'm kidding – there's nothing written there. Careful, you'll drop it!'

Jaz, face like a thundercloud, set the head a little too heavily on the shelf. 'If you aren't going to take this seriously –'

'I am! I am! Okay, I'm being completely serious now. Trust me, that head is not ancient. It's bonded stone – powdered stone mixed with resin and poured into a mould. My dad's an art teacher, so I know all about this stuff. It's just a cheap modern copy of an ancient Greek head.' She glanced at Jaz, then added, 'Or an ancient Roman head.'

Chapter Two

'Well ... I guess it's good that it isn't *really* valuable,' said Jaz, slightly mollified. 'Given that you nearly made me *drop it*. Still, it must have been significant to Dr Huxley.'

'Who's – Oh, right, the guy who collected all this stuff.'

'What do you think comes next?' said Jaz. 'After ancient times was, um ... the Middle Ages?'

They studied the objects on the table.

'How about this little painting?' said Rosy. 'It's got that flat medieval look about it.' The figure had been painted onto a piece of dark wood in bright colours, with his halo highlighted in gold leaf. 'I think it's a religious icon.'

'Is it a picture of Jesus?'

'I'm not sure.' Rosy looked at it closely. It was a very small painting, about the size of Rosy's palm. 'He seems to be buried up to his waist in a big pot of dirt. Did that ever happen to Jesus?'

'No idea,' said Jaz. 'My family's Sikh – I don't go to church.' Then she gasped. 'Church! The Crypt! I forgot the key to the Crypt!' In response to Rosy's unspoken question, she babbled, 'There's a bathroom in there that my dad uses during the day, but it's locked and he can't get in and he'll wonder where I've got to! I'll be right back!' Then she raced off.

Shrugging, Rosy returned her attention to the little painting. There was writing along one edge, but the letters were too tiny to decipher. 'Let's just call him *Random Medieval Saint* for the moment,' she told herself, propping the painting against the back of the shelf. 'Now, what's next?'

The skeleton illustration with the Latin captions? Or the yellowing fragments of old English text? But wait ... *was* that English?

She chose a line at random and read: 'Two of the worft patients, with the tendons in the ham rigid, (a fymptom none of the reft had), were put under a courfe of feawater.'

What on Earth did *that* mean? Still, Latin had to be older than English – even Ye Olde Incomprehensible English – so she sat the framed skeleton drawing beside Random Medieval Saint.

The next two objects were easy – the two mahogany boxes, numbered five and six, containing the flask of liquid and the weird tin contraption. She arranged them on the middle shelf with their lids thrown back. She was pondering her next move when Jaz rushed back in.

'What did you put next?' she gasped. 'Oh, the skeleton picture. I don't suppose you know what any of those words say?'

'No,' said Rosy. 'I wish I *could* read them. But we can't do Latin at our school till Year Eleven.'

'Your school offers *Latin*? What school do you go to?'

'Blue Mountains Ladies' College,' said Rosy. 'But not because we're rich or anything. It's only because Dad's the head of the art department there and Gabrielle – that's his partner – teaches ceramics, so we get a big discount on the fees. If I went to the state high school down the mountains, I'd have to spend hours on the bus each day. What school do you go to?'

'Parkerville High,' said Jaz.

'Oh,' said Rosy, because Parkerville High was famous. 'Okay.'

'It's not as bad as they made it sound on the news,' said Jaz, rather defensively. 'Most of those boys with knives weren't even students. The one who got stabbed wasn't even inside the school grounds.'

'Well, that's ... good.' Rosy cast around for a way to change the subject. 'Hey, what language did you do last year? We did French. It was excellent! If I go to Paris, I'll be able to count to twenty and ask the way to the Louvre and order a ham and cheese croissant.'

'We were supposed to do Indonesian,' said Jaz gloomily. 'But the teacher resigned in the first week, so we just did worksheets by ourselves for the rest of the term.'

'Still, I bet you'll get a new teacher this year,' said Rosy. 'And you probably have much better uniforms than we do. We have to wear stupid straw hats with elastic that cuts into your chin and you're not allowed to take your blazer off, ever, not even when it's boiling hot and everyone's keeling over from sunstroke.'

Jaz gave a faint smile. 'Anyway,' she said, and turned back to the table. 'What's next? I suppose it's these fragments of ... What *is* this?'

'It's either a secret code or just really old English,' said Rosy. 'But I think it's number seven.'

'Then ... maybe this other head?' said Jaz.

'The *creepy* head,' said Rosy, with a melodramatic shudder.

'If it weren't for the writing all over it,' Jaz mused aloud, 'it'd look like a head from one of those old china dolls.'

'The kind that comes to life in the middle of the night and goes around strangling people in their beds,' said Rosy. 'And what's with the big gaping hole in its throat?'

'Secretiveness. Friendship. Individuality,' said Jaz. She was reading the words written on the head. 'Hope. Mirth. Amativeness. What's amativeness?'

'Who knows? Just stick that thing in the cabinet before it starts casting spells on us.'

'Cautiousness,' murmured Jaz, setting it on the bottom shelf. The face stared blindly in Rosy's direction, a serene smile playing over its features.

'You know,' said Rosy, frowning back at it, 'there's something familiar about that head. I'm sure I've seen something like it before …'

Jaz waited, her dark eyebrows inching up her forehead.

Rosy shook her head. 'No, it'll probably come to me later. The box of Aspro next, I think, because the label looks so old-fashioned. It must be a hundred years old. Much older than the smallpox vaccine, anyway.'

'What about this?' said Jaz, flipping open the little leather case.

'Oh, yeah. Hmm, I thought it was a medal.'

'No, it's something in a little round frame. A portrait?'

Chapter Two

'Ugh!' said Rosy, looking closer. 'It's all *mouldy*. Water must have got under the glass. Now the paper's ruined and we'll never know what it was … Unless there's something written on the leather case?'

'Afraid not,' said Jaz, after further scrutiny.

'Can we chuck it out?'

'No,' said Jaz firmly. 'It's part of Dr Huxley's collection.' She sat the open case beside the Aspro packet, then placed the smallpox vaccine next to them.

'What I want to know,' said Rosy, 'is why a vaccine is labelled "NOT FOR INJECTION". What *else* would you do with a vaccine?'

'At least that one's going to be easy to research,' said Jaz. 'It's the only thing where we'll know exactly what to type into Google.'

'And last of all, the metal spiral,' said Rosy. 'Because it's obviously the most modern.'

'Hang on, we forgot this yellow stone,' said Jaz. She held it up to the light. 'It's got something inside it. A twig or something, with a little leaf attached.'

'Cool,' said Rosy, examining it. She placed it on its blue velvet square on the bottom shelf, next to the metal spiral, and Jaz picked up the notebook and pen she'd brought back with her.

'I'm going to write down a description of each item,' she announced.

'And I'll run downstairs and get my camera so we can have photos *and* descriptions,' said Rosy, 'for when we can't get access to the cabinet. I mean, this room's locked most of the time, isn't it?'

'Excellent plan,' said Jaz, and they proceeded to carry it out.

'Now let's go down to Mum's flat so we can look at these photos,' Rosy said, tossing the last of the pellets back into the carton. 'It's lucky I decided to bring Methuselah with me on holidays.'

Methuselah was Rosy's laptop computer. She'd inherited him from her mum six years ago, which made him about a thousand years old in computer age. His battery didn't work properly, so he had to be plugged into a power point, and he lapsed into sulky fits if Rosy typed too quickly or opened more than one program at a time. However, on this occasion, she managed to transfer all the photos from her camera to his hard drive without him grumbling too much.

'I'll print out the best photo for each object,' said Rosy. 'Then you can have copies to put in your notebook.'

Jaz glanced up from the sofa, where she'd been poring over her notes. 'Good, because I'll need to take all this home to do extra work on it each evening. We've only got two weeks. That's hardly any time at all, when you consider –'

'Will you stop *fussing*?' said Rosy. 'Do something useful and stand next to the printer to catch the pages.'

She'd plugged Methuselah into her mum's little printer, which was currently grinding out an image of the ancient Egyptian eye. Jaz had insisted they do everything in the correct sequence, even printing out photos.

'Dr Huxley must have put all these things in order for a reason,' Jaz said, as Rosy coaxed Methuselah along. 'Anyway, it makes sense for us to research them from oldest to newest, so we're working through history.'

The printer dropped a second page into Jaz's waiting hands, then began labouring away at image number three.

'We just need to figure out what his theme was,' mused Jaz.

'Huh?' said Rosy, distracted by the printer's blinking red light.

'Well, collections have themes, don't they? They're not just random objects – they're connected, they *mean* something. All these objects must be about an idea or a subject or – What? What's wrong?'

'Nothing. The printer's run out of ink, that's all ... Oh, and there don't seem to be any spare ink cartridges.'

Then Methuselah made an angry spluttering noise and went blank. Jaz looked even more alarmed.

'Don't worry,' said Rosy. 'He does that sometimes. I think he gets annoyed if no one's paying attention to him. Or he might have overheated ... Hey, I know what! Let's go for a walk and buy another ink cartridge. By the time we get back, Methuselah might be in a better mood. Maybe he'll even let us connect to the internet.' She stood up and brushed off her hands. 'And then –' she narrowed her eyes '– we can begin solving the strange and mysterious enigma of Dr Huxley's bequest.'

CHAPTER THREE

'I have no special talents. I am only passionately curious.'
~ Albert Einstein

It was barely halfway through the morning and already the air was a shimmering heat haze and the road was melting into sticky black puddles. When Jaz had told her father where they were going, he'd insisted that Rosy put on a sunhat too and now she was glad she'd run back to her room to fetch it. She flipped up its brim to squint into the distance, wishing she'd also remembered to grab her sunglasses.

'We have to go to my mum's office first,' she told Jaz, 'so I can borrow some money and her staff discount card. Her meeting must be over by now.'

'Which way?' asked Jaz.

'Left,' said Rosy decisively, leading them towards a lofty edifice of neo-Gothic sandstone. They passed under a clock tower, through an ivy-smothered archway and found themselves in a quadrangle of manicured lawn neatly divided by flagstone paths. The surrounding buildings featured turrets and parapets, ornate stained-glass windows and a veritable menagerie of gargoyles and grotesques. The girls stared around, feeling rather dazed. Although perhaps that was just from the heat.

'Actually,' said Rosy, 'I think we were supposed to go right, not left. I never *usually* get lost. I have an excellent sense of direction. It must be sunstroke. Let's go this way.'

They walked along some shady cloisters and through a doorway into a vestibule presided over by an ancient marble Roman on a pedestal. Rosy had her head tilted back at a dizzying angle, admiring the elaborate carvings of the vaulted stone ceiling, when she became aware that Jaz was tugging on her sleeve.

'What?' said Rosy.

Jaz silently pointed to a nearby sign, which declared, 'Secrets of the Mummies Revealed! Now open. Admission is free.'

Below this writing was a picture of an Egyptian coffin decorated in vivid colours. The girls peered past the sign to a set of glass doors labelled: 'THE NICHOLSON MUSEUM'.

'Obviously, this is where I was leading us all along,' said Rosy. 'So we could go in and check out their ancient Egyptian artefacts and find out what our eye ornament is supposed to be.'

Jaz snorted, then stalked through the doors.

The first thing Rosy noticed (apart from the deliciously cool air conditioning) was a glass case containing the very same coffin depicted on the sign. 'Isn't this amazing?' she whispered. They were the only people in sight, but it was the sort of place where

Chapter Three

you spoke in hushed, respectful tones. 'Look at the decorations on it!'

'Can you see any eye shapes?' asked Jaz.

'There's one here, in the hieroglyphics on the bottom. And another one. And one over here – Wait, where are you going?'

Jaz had strolled away into the adjacent room and was scrutinising the contents of a display table. A few minutes later, Rosy heard a hiss and looked up to see Jaz making urgent beckoning motions. Rosy reluctantly abandoned the beautiful coffin and went over.

'I've found it!' Jaz whispered, pointing to a familiar-looking blue-green ornament. 'The Eye of Horus!'

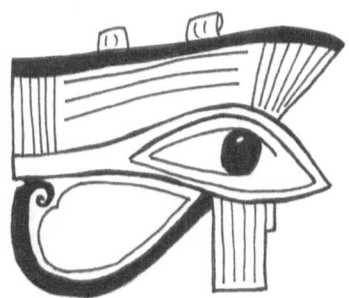

'Oh,' said Rosy. 'Who's Horus?'

'It doesn't say.' Jaz studied the tag beside the object. 'It's also called a *wedjat*-eye amulet and it's dated between 1550 BC and AD 395.'

'I think *our* eye is nicer,' said Rosy. 'It's got better carvings and more colours. It's probably older, too.'

Jaz was busy copying down the information in her notebook. 'I wish they'd said what it was *for*. Never mind, we can look it up when we get back. See if you can find anything else related to Horus.'

Rosy checked out various display shelves without success, then turned to the glass case behind her. It contained a small figure wrapped in linen bandages. She read out the accompanying information: '"The mummy of the boy Horus". Wow, he must have been a pretty famous kid, if they named amulets after his eye.'

'Or there was some Egyptian god called Horus, and both the boy and the amulets were named after the god,' said Jaz, coming to stand beside Rosy. 'Oh, he was only five or six years old. Look, they did CT scans of his head and found his baby teeth.'

'What!' said Rosy, taking a step back. 'Wait, this is the *actual* dead boy? Right here, inside these bandages?'

'You *have* heard of mummies, right?' said Jaz. 'The embalmed-body, wrapped-in-bandages, preserved-in-the-sands-of-Egypt kind?'

'Of course I have!' said Rosy. 'But I thought this was just a model, to show what the actual mummy looked like!'

'This is a university museum. That body is real. And about two thousand years old.'

'Jaz, it's a *dead child*!'

'Well, if that bothers you, you probably shouldn't look at that cabinet in the corner.'

Naturally, Rosy had to go over and look at it. 'Ugh!' She felt slightly sick, but she couldn't pull her gaze away from it. There was a blackened mummified hand in an old Arnott's biscuit tin, a mummified head with

Chapter Three

a gold disc lodged inside one eye socket, and a pair of tiny mummified legs, the bones and sinews visible inside leathery, orange-brown skin, the toes curled up, a wafer-thin grey toenail still clinging to the ancient flesh.

'It says here they used to grind up mummified bodies for medicine,' said Jaz. 'As treatment for "abscesses, concussion, paralysis, coughs, nausea and ulcers". Not the ancient Egyptians, but other people, later on.'

'*Treatment* for nausea?' said Rosy. 'Swallowing ground-up bits of mummies would definitely *cause* nausea. It's bad enough looking at them. Go on, admit it, even *you* think that mummified head is creepy.'

'It is a bit disturbing,' Jaz agreed. 'Not because it's dead. Just because it's a face.'

'It's like something out of a horror movie,' said Rosy. 'The stained, unravelling bandages. The yellow teeth, bared in an infernal grimace. The staring, hollow eyes –'

The girls gazed into the glass-fronted cabinet and became aware, at exactly the same moment, that a tall pale figure was reflected in the glass, looming up behind them.

'AARRGGHH!' they screamed, whirling around.

'Oh, I didn't mean to startle you,' said the young woman wearing a long white shirt and an apologetic expression. 'It's just that I saw you taking notes, so I wondered if you had any questions. I'm Naomi, one of the guides here.'

Jaz released her grip on Rosy's arm, took a step sideways and cleared her throat. 'Could you tell us about the Eye of Horus, please?' she said, hastily gathering up the remnants of her dignity.

'Ah, were you looking at our *wedjat* eye?' said Naomi. 'That's one of my favourites! Well, Horus was an Egyptian god of the sky, usually depicted as a man with the head of a falcon. He had his left eye gouged out when he was fighting with Seth, the god of chaos, but the goddess Hathor healed it. The eye of Horus – injured, then healed – represented the waxing and waning of the moon each month. Then Horus gave his eye to Osiris, his dead father, to bring him back to life, so the *wedjat* eye was also a symbol of regeneration. *Wedjat* means "whole" or "restored", so *wedjat*-eye amulets were very popular, for both the living and the dead. If you unwrap a mummy, you'll often find *wedjat*-eye amulets among the bandages.'

'Could they be worn as necklaces?' asked Rosy, while Jaz searched through her notebook for the photo of Dr Huxley's Egyptian ornament.

'Oh, yes,' said Naomi. 'As necklaces or rings.' She examined the page that Jaz held out. 'Yes, that's a *wedjat* eye. See the spiral and that line below the eye? They're like the markings around a falcon's eye.'

'Do you think our amulet might be really *rare* and *valuable*?' asked Rosy.

'Well, there are a lot of *wedjat*-eye amulets around,' said Naomi. Rosy's face fell. 'Although,' Naomi added quickly, 'this looks like a particularly nice example of one. I've seen something similar in the British Museum's collection. Third Intermediate Period, I think – that's about 1000 BC. Oh, and that blue-green colour is also a symbol of regeneration.'

'So the Egyptians believed these eye amulets had *healing powers*?' said Jaz. She gave Rosy a significant look, involving a lot of eyebrow action. Unfortunately, Rosy was not fluent in this particular dialect of Eyebrow Language, so she had no idea what Jaz was getting at.

'Ooh, I'm so glad you asked that!' Naomi beamed at them. She lowered her voice. 'Sorry, I'm writing my thesis on the Edwin Smith and Ebers papyri – they're the ancient Egyptian versions of medical textbooks – so I love it when I get a chance to talk about this stuff.'

'A thesis is a very long essay that PhD students write about their research,' Jaz told Rosy.

'I *know* that,' said Rosy, rolling her eyes.

'Anyway,' said Naomi hastily, 'the Egyptians believed that angry gods or evil forces caused illness, so people used a lot of magical remedies, like incantations and amulets. Priests or magicians often treated the sick. Sick people would visit healing statues in the temples or drink water that had been poured over stone columns engraved with spells.'

'But there were doctors as well?' said Jaz.

'Yes, ancient Egypt was famous for its skilled physicians and surgeons. They had a huge influence on the Greeks and Romans. The Egyptians developed ointments, pills, lozenges, eye drops, mouthwashes, inhalations, poultices … and of course, they were experts at applying bandages.'

They all looked at the neatly wrapped figure of little Horus.

'They used honey or soap to stop the linen sticking to wounds,' Naomi went on. 'They even made special adhesive bandages to draw together the edges of gaping wounds, so they healed faster.'

'So they invented Band-Aids!' said Rosy, and Naomi nodded enthusiastically.

'What were their medicines like?' asked Jaz.

'Well, some of their treatments were quite sensible. They knew that opium extracted from poppies would relieve pain, for instance, and that honey helped soothe a cough. They covered infected wounds with willow leaves – and now we know that willow is a natural source of aspirin, which treats fever. But most of their practices seem a little ... er, strange to us now. For example, if a child was having teething problems, the mother and the child had to eat a cooked mouse, then the mouse bones were put in a linen bag tied with seven knots and worn around the child's neck. The Egyptians were very keen on using mice. I remember one treatment for clogged-up ears – head of rodent, mixed with gall bladder of goat, shell of tortoise and fleawort.'

'I'm not even going to *ask* what fleawort is,' said Rosy. She was sure it was something disgusting.

'Yes, they certainly used some odd ingredients. Mud, sand, ash, beer, rotten wood, crocodile dung ... Of course, the Egyptians had good reason to worry about illness. Up to half of their babies died before their first birthday and only a few adults lived past the age of thirty-five. We have evidence they suffered from all sorts of diseases – smallpox, malaria, even tapeworms and rotten teeth. Have you seen the CT scans of this adult mummy?'

She led them over to the wall, where some black-and-white images of a skull were clipped to a light box.

'See the huge holes in his teeth and jaw? Poor man, he must have been in agony. That might even have been the reason he died. The sand got into their food, you see, and ground away the enamel on their teeth, so they had lots of dental infections.'

'Is this the mummy from that beautiful coffin?' asked Rosy.

'Ah. Well, yes and no,' said Naomi. 'The writing on the coffin shows it belongs to a priest called Padiashaikhet, who lived around 700 BC. We thought the mummy inside was him, too, but it was carbon-dated last year and that told us the body was actually from about AD 100, eight hundred years after the coffin was made. Probably the dealer who owned the empty coffin thought it would be more valuable with a mummy inside, so he found some random mummy, stuck it in the coffin and sold the whole set to the collector who donated it to the university.'

'So all this time, you were certain it was one thing,' said Jaz, in rather accusing tones, 'and you turned out to be completely *wrong*.'

'But that's the beauty of science,' said Naomi, smiling at her. 'New tests come along and we learn new facts, then we have to change our ideas.'

'Hmm,' said Jaz. Rosy could already tell Jaz was the sort of person who preferred things to stay stuck down firmly where they'd been placed and not wobble about in unpredictable ways.

They heard the soft *whump* of the museum doors and Naomi looked around. 'There's someone at the desk,' she said. 'I have to go – but come and ask if you have any more questions.'

'No, this has been excellent,' said Rosy. 'Thanks for all your help.'

'Yes, thank you very much,' said Jaz, although she was fiddling with her pen and didn't look up.

'Okay, so what was all that about?' Rosy demanded, once the two girls were back outside. 'That eyebrow thing?'

'What?' said Jaz. She frowned, pulled her hat from her waistband and jammed it back on her head. 'It must be thirty-five degrees out here. We should've brought water bottles with us.'

'You *know*. When Naomi was explaining about the amulet!'

'We'll probably collapse from dehydration before we ever find your mum's office.'

'There's a bubbler over there,' said Rosy. 'Then we can – Hey, that's the library! I know exactly where we are now! All we have to do is turn right and follow that path.'

They crossed the road and took it in turns to gulp down mouthfuls of water, which was lovely and cold once the bubbler had run for a minute.

Chapter Three

'Anyway,' said Rosy, standing up and wiping her chin, 'you still haven't answered my question. Did you figure out something to do with our objects? Have you worked out how they're all connected?'

'Weren't you *listening* to what Naomi said?'

'Yes! But what did that have to do with Dr Huxley?'

Jaz sighed. 'Well, isn't it *obvious*?' Then she turned and walked off.

She was so annoying that Rosy refused to speak to her until they'd followed the path all the way to City Road and were climbing the steps to the footbridge. Rosy figured Jaz had been sufficiently punished by then. Also, Rosy had just thought of a hypothesis and wanted to discuss it.

CHAPTER FOUR

'The scientific mind does not so much provide the right answers as ask the right questions.'
~ Claude Lévi-Strauss

'You,' Rosy said to Jaz, 'must be an only child.'

Jaz, who'd clearly been lost in her own thoughts – and, in fact, had given no indication that she realised she *was* being punished – gave Rosy a startled, sideways look. 'What?'

'That's my hypothesis,' said Rosy. 'I thought it up just now. A hypothesis is an idea that explains something.'

'I *know* what a hypothesis is,' Jaz huffed. 'Anyway, there's no point having a hypothesis unless you can back it up with evidence.'

'I have heaps of evidence that you're an only child,' Rosy said, 'thanks to my amazing powers of observation. For instance, I noticed what your dad said when you told him where we were going. He told you to use the footbridge if we needed to cross City Road.'

'So?'

'So, he's worried about your safety,' Rosy said. 'Because you're an only child.'

'What kind of evidence is that?' said Jaz. 'He'd still be worried about me getting run over if I had brothers or sisters. This road is really busy. And look, that car just drove through a red light!'

'Oh, that's not my only evidence.' Rosy sauntered along the footbridge and peered down at the traffic. 'You show many other signs of being an only child. *Obvious* signs.'

Jaz refused to bite. 'Do we go down these stairs?'

'No, along here,' said Rosy. 'Yes, anyway, I know all about being an only child, because I used to be one too, for years and years. But then Gabrielle had Reuben, so now I have a little brother. He's gone with Dad and Gabrielle to visit her parents up north, while I'm staying with my mum.'

'Well, as it happens,' said Jaz, 'I *don't* have any brothers or sisters. But we live with my aunt and uncle and I have lots of cousins, so that's practically the same thing.'

'How many cousins?' asked Rosy with interest.

'Twenty-three.'

'All in the one house?'

'*No*, of course not,' said Jaz. 'Only three in our house. But my dad has three brothers and two sisters, and they all have kids.'

'Cool,' said Rosy. 'I've only got two cousins and I hardly ever see them because they live in Perth. Here we are.'

The walkway had brought them to a massive block of concrete that had been clad in brown pebble

Chapter Four

dash and wedged into a grassy slope. 'DEPARTMENTS OF BIOCHEMISTRY AND MICROBIOLOGY,' announced the sign above its glass doors. But when they reached the office labelled 'DR ALISON RADFORD', they found a lanky young man sitting at her desk, tapping away at a laptop.

'Oh, hi,' he said, glancing up. 'You just missed your mum. She rang your flat about five minutes ago and left a message, said she wouldn't be back for lunch. She has another meeting.' He pointed at the ceiling. 'Upstairs. With the big cheese.'

Rosy sighed. 'Great. I'd better leave her a note, then. Can I borrow your pen, Jaz? And some paper? This is Marcus, by the way. He's one of Mum's post-graduate students. Marcus, Jaz.'

'Hail,' said Marcus.

'Hello,' said Jaz, eyeing his T-shirt. It was green with large black letters that said, 'NINJA', and then, in smaller letters below this, 'CLEVERLY DISGUISED AS A MICROBIOLOGIST'.

'You know,' said Rosy, writing away in the back of Jaz's notebook, 'this could all have been avoided if I was allowed to have my own phone. Mum could have called me directly.'

'My dad says I can't have my own phone till I start Year Nine,' said Jaz glumly. 'And that's a whole year away. Until then, I have to share with my cousin.'

'My dad says I can't have one till I'm old enough to get a job and pay all the phone bills myself,' said Rosy. 'And Gabrielle thinks mobile phones cause brain cancer, so I shouldn't be allowed one anyway. It's so unfair.'

'Yes, what a terrible violation of your human rights,' said Marcus. 'Quick, call the International Court of Justice. Oh, wait, you can't, you don't have a phone.'

'Just ignore him,' Rosy advised Jaz. 'There. I've asked Mum to buy more printer cartridges on her way back.'

'Used up all your mum's printer ink?' said Marcus. 'Printing out photos of your favourite teenybopper idols, no doubt.'

'*Teenybopper?*' said Rosy, forgetting her own advice. 'What are you, seventy years old? And for your information, Jaz and I happen to be working on a very important investigation.'

She handed Jaz her notebook back, but a loose paper had worked itself free and drifted down to land beside one of Marcus's oversized purple sneakers. He stooped to retrieve the paper.

'I see,' he said, holding the photo out to Jaz. 'An important investigation into Egyptian healing amulets, apparently.'

Jaz froze, her arm outstretched.

'You know about the Eye of Horus?' said Rosy.

'I know many things, Grasshopper,' said Marcus. 'Many, *many* things.'

The girls exchanged glances.

'Show him the next photo,' ordered Rosy. Jaz pulled out the image of the old bearded man and held it up.

'Do you recognise this person?' Rosy said to Marcus.

Chapter Four

'Sure. That's Hippocrates,' said Marcus.

'Hip-oc-ruh-teez,' Rosy repeated slowly, so she'd remember it. 'How do you *know* that?'

'Because my dad has one of those in his consulting rooms,' said Marcus. 'He's a cardiologist. My dad, that is, not Hippocrates. I don't think the ancient Greeks knew all that much about heart surgery.'

'This old man is from ancient *Greece*?' said Rosy, unable to resist shooting Jaz a told-you-so look. But Jaz didn't even notice.

'Wait,' Jaz said. 'This is Hippocrates? You mean, like the Hippocratic oath?'

'That's the one,' said Marcus.

'That's the oath that doctors take,' said Jaz, turning to Rosy.

'Doctors!' cried Rosy. 'Healing! Medicine! That's it. *That's* the connection!'

'I *told* you it was obvious,' said Jaz, scribbling in her notebook.

'It wasn't obvious *then*,' said Rosy in exasperation. 'You only had one piece of evidence. Now we've got two.'

'More than two,' countered Jaz. 'The vaccine. The Aspro box. The skeleton.'

'Well, if you've solved your very important case ...' said Marcus, flapping a hand at the door.

'Oh, yeah, sorry,' said Rosy. 'We're going now. And thanks!'

'No worries,' he said. 'See you later, Sherlock and Dr Watson.'

Rosy and Jaz argued most of the way back to New College about which one of them was Sherlock and which was Watson.

By the time they arrived, all they'd managed to agree upon was that they were both starving. Jaz had brought some sort of delicious-smelling vegetable curry from home, which she heated up in the kitchen microwave, while Rosy made herself a cheese, beetroot and lettuce sandwich at the counter. Then they carried their plates into the refectory, where they settled at the end of one of the long wooden tables so that Rosy could plug Methuselah into the wall. Fortunately, he was in a cooperative mood and the refectory had excellent wi-fi.

'Hippocrates,' said Rosy, between bites of her sandwich. 'Here he is. The Father of Medicine. Born in about 460 BC in Greece. Wrote at least sixty medical texts – no, wait, they were probably written by his students, not him. Anyway, he believed that diseases *weren't* caused by the gods, but by people's lifestyles.'

'Well, that's an advance on the ancient Egyptians,' said Jaz.

'He also thought it was important to figure out the cause of a disease. "It is not sufficient to learn simply that cheese is a bad food, as it gives a pain to one who eats a surfeit of it; we must know what the pain is, the reasons for it, and which constituent of man is harmfully affected."' Rosy put down the remainder of her sandwich and stared at it. 'Cheese is a bad food?'

'Of course it isn't,' said Jaz. 'It's full of calcium. Anyway, he only said a *surfeit* of cheese was bad. One slice is not a surfeit. Go on.'

'Two slices, actually, but okay. Um ... Hippocrates worked out that diseases could be either *acute*, which means short but severe, or *chronic*, which means they go on and on. And he thought that for every disease, there was a crisis point, and after that, the patient would either die or get better. Or the patient might get better, then have a relapse and die.'

'Well, how is *that* useful to know?' said Jaz. 'Naturally, if you're sick, you either get better or you die!'

'Yeah, that was a big part of his philosophy, too. Nature, I mean. He reckoned doctors should stand back and let Nature do the healing. The doctor's job was mostly to keep patients clean and make them rest in bed.'

'No medicine?'

'Not usually. It was more about diet – like, lots of barley water and honey if someone had a fever. Oh, and here's what he thought caused diseases. People would get sick if they had an imbalance of the four humours, which were black bile, yellow bile, blood and phlegm. Gross. I'm glad I've finished eating.' Rosy pushed her plate away.

'That sounds a lot like traditional Indian Ayurvedic medicine,' said Jaz. 'One of my aunties is really into that. But I think that only has three humours.'

'Anyway, Hippocrates said that to get better, you basically had to wait for Nature to get rid of your excess phlegm, or bile, or whatever.'

'He must have done more than that to become the Father of Medicine. Look up the Hippocratic oath.'

'Okay, here it is. *I swear by Apollo the Healer, and by Asclepius and Hygieia and Panacea and all the gods and goddesses –*'

'I thought he didn't believe in gods and goddesses.'

'He did, he just didn't think they caused diseases. Hey, wait – Hygieia! That's probably where we get the word "hygiene". Because to be healthy, you need to be hygienic! And you know, "panacea" means "a cure-all". I wonder if Asclepius is related to medicine, too ... Yes! Asclepius, the god of physicians, was usually shown holding a staff and a snake, because snakes shed their skin, which is a symbol of regeneration. And that's why modern doctors have a stick with a snake twisted around it as their symbol. Cool. Anyway, the oath goes on: *To hold him who has taught me this art as equal to my parents –*'

'Maybe you could just paraphrase,' said Jaz.

'Okay. Um, respect your teacher and teach other students what you know, but only if they've taken this oath. Do no harm. Don't hand out deadly medicines. Don't do any surgery – Wow, I wonder if Marcus's dad has actually *read* this oath. Oh, it just means doctors should leave surgery to specialist surgeons. Okay. Treat patients kindly. Don't take advantage of them. Don't gossip about them. That's about it.'

Chapter Four

'So Hippocrates was the first to say that doctors should be professional and ethical.'

Rosy shrugged. 'I don't know about the *first*, but it says here he had lots of rules for how doctors should behave, even about how long their fingernails should be. Doctors had to be clean and honest and serious. They had to observe patients' symptoms carefully, and ask about their lifestyle, and keep detailed medical records and – Oh, Methuselah!'

'What's he doing?'

'He flickered at me. He needs a break, I think. Have you finished eating? Let's go up to my room.'

They stacked their plates in the dishwasher, grabbed some apples from the fruit bowl and headed upstairs. As Alison's flat contained only one bed and her sofa wasn't very comfortable, Rosy was allowed to sleep in a student's room, and she'd chosen one tucked away in a corner of the top floor.

'Isn't this brilliant?' said Rosy, throwing open the door to a small room with stone walls and bare wooden floorboards. 'It's like living in a castle. And look, I've got my very own gargoyle!' She climbed onto the desk, pushed open the diamond-paned window and pointed to the stone demon clinging to the outside wall. One of his horns was broken and moss oozed from his nostrils, but he had a very appealing grin. 'And I can stay here all holidays, Mum said, unless they need the room for conference visitors or something, but they probably won't, because grown-ups don't want to climb all those stairs. Have a seat … Oh, just chuck all those clothes on the bed.' Rosy plugged Methuselah in and his screen lit up at once. 'Yes! Okay, so where were we?'

'In ancient Greece,' said Jaz, opening her notebook and uncapping her pen.

'Whenever *I* think of ancient Greece,' said Rosy, while they waited for Methuselah to connect to the internet, 'I picture that fresco by Raphael, with all the Greek philosophers standing about in their robes, chatting to each other. You know, the one with Socrates and Plato and Aristotle and um ... Actually, they're the only Greek philosophers I know.'

'Were any of them doctors?'

'I think Aristotle might have been. Let me check ... Yes, he was! Sort of. Born in 384 BC, studied medicine, but was also an expert in zoology, physics, poetry, logic, politics and ... yeah, basically everything. He's known as the Father of Science because he said theories should be based on facts, and facts came from observing the world. If you found a new fact that went against your theory, he reckoned you should either change your theory or come up with a new one. He also discovered the four basic qualities, which were hot, cold, wet and dry. Plus, he studied animals to find out how human bodies worked and um ... got a few things wrong.'

Jaz frowned. 'Such as?'

'Such as, he reckoned men had more teeth than women. And he saw the heart beating and decided it controlled everything in the body – breathing, movement, sensation, the lot. It's really the brain that does that, but Aristotle thought the brain was mostly there to cool the blood down. And he said the heart had three chambers, instead of four, and he thought veins and arteries were the same thing. Oh, well, nobody's perfect. Anyway, animal bodies are probably different to human bodies.'

'He should have studied dead humans, then,' said Jaz.

'He couldn't,' said Rosy, 'because it says here that cutting up dead people was forbidden in ancient Greece. Hang on, Herophilus and Erasistratus did cut up dead people, but they were about fifty years after Aristotle. No, wait – they cut up *living* people! Condemned criminals! And they did horrible experiments on live pigs, too! Oh, this is *so* disgusting – I'm not reading any more of this.'

Jaz pulled Methuselah towards her. 'But look, they discovered something really important,' she pointed out. 'They realised that nerves lead from your brain and spinal cord to your arms and legs, and that lets you move and feel sensation. And Herophilus saw that the heart pumped blood through veins and arteries, but that only arteries had a pulse. He even worked out a way of diagnosing diseases based on how weak or slow or irregular the patient's pulse was.'

'Hello? Are you forgetting he worked that out by CUTTING OPEN PEOPLE WHILE THEY WERE STILL ALIVE?'

'But they were criminals. They'd already been sentenced to death. They were going to die anyway, and at least this way, they helped doctors understand more about how bodies work.'

'I bet you wouldn't feel that way if *you* were a condemned criminal,' said Rosy. 'Or one of those poor innocent pigs. Have we finished with the ancient Greeks now?'

'We could move on to the ancient Romans,' said Jaz. 'It might help us work out Dr Huxley's next object ... Except didn't you think that one was from the Middle Ages?'

'If we keep going through history, we'll end up in the Middle Ages sooner or later,' said Rosy.

'Yes, but we've got thirteen objects to figure out and only two weeks to –'

'Don't you want to do this properly?' asked Rosy.

'Yes! But –'

'Ancient Romans it is,' said Rosy, taking back Methuselah. 'And I hope they're nicer than the Greeks.'

Jaz sighed. 'Well, considering they used to throw Christians to the lions and make gladiators fight to the death in the Colosseum and –'

'Gladiators!' cried Rosy. 'Listen to this! Ancient Romans with epilepsy used to *suck blood* from the wounds of gladiators! They reckoned it was a "most effectual cure for their disease"! Jaz, these people were VAMPIRES!'

'I'm sure *some* of the Romans had sensible ideas,' said Jaz, scanning the screen. 'Yes, look, here's Celsus. He said that after surgery, doctors should watch patients carefully for the four signs of inflammation, which were heat, redness, pain and swelling. See, that's exactly what doctors do now. But who's Galen?

Chapter Four

They keep mentioning his name. He's supposed to be the most important person in Roman medicine.'

Rosy tapped at the keyboard for a moment. 'Galen of Pergamon. Born AD 129 to rich Greek parents, travelled widely, learned all about Egyptian, Indian and African medicine. Was appointed physician to the gladiators and found this very useful because their wounds were "windows into the body". Did lots of revolting public experiments on live pigs and apes, which impressed everyone so much that the Romans appointed him personal physician to the emperor ... You know what? I think the Romans were actually *worse* than the Greeks.'

Jaz nudged Rosy aside and read on. 'Galen combined Hippocrates' four humours and Aristotle's four basic qualities with other factors such as weather and diet, and said all of these influenced a person's health. For instance, eating cold food in winter would produce an excess of phlegm and cause cold diseases. Each person also had a particular temperament, based on which humour they had too much of. Their temperament would make them susceptible to certain diseases and affect their behaviour.'

'Temperament? Is that the same as personality?' asked Rosy.

'I guess so,' said Jaz. 'The four main temperaments were sanguine, choleric, melancholic and phlegmatic. Sanguine people were sociable, confident, sensitive and creative –'

'Hey, that's me!' said Rosy.

'They could also be impulsive, forgetful and chronically late,' said Jaz pointedly.

'Yeah, well, it says here that *choleric* people are ambitious and dominating.' Rosy poked her finger at the screen. 'That's just a fancy way of saying they're *bossy*. Plus, they have mood swings.'

'It also says they're energetic and *highly organised*,' said Jaz.

'Although you could be melancholic,' said Rosy. 'They're perfectionists who worry too much.'

'But it says they're also thoughtful, independent and reliable.' Jaz paused for a moment. 'Hmm, I think my dad's melancholic.'

'My dad's definitely phlegmatic,' said Rosy. 'Quiet, relaxed, kind and curious. Ha, I'm going to have to tell him he's cold and moist and has an excess of phlegm! But, hang on. Galen reckoned your personality showed what sort of diseases you'd get – but could he actually do anything once you *did* get sick? Apart from telling you to avoid cold foods in winter?'

Jaz scrolled down the page. 'Diseases were due to excess humours building up in the body, causing decay, heat and fever,' she read. 'Galen's preferred treatment was bloodletting.'

'Does "bloodletting" mean what I think it means?' Rosy scrunched up her face.

'Yes, if you thought it meant cutting open a vein and letting out blood. Lots and lots of blood. Until the patient fainted.'

'Oh, I'm sure that would have helped the patient. NOT.'

Chapter Four

'Galen was convinced he was right. "It is I, and I alone, who have revealed the true path of medicine." He developed all these complicated rules about which vein to use and how much blood to let out ... Actually, you didn't even have to be sick for him to recommend bloodletting. He thought it also prevented fevers in healthy people.'

'I'm so glad I don't live in ancient Rome,' said Rosy.

'But Galen did figure out a lot about anatomy, including how blood circulates around the body,' said Jaz. 'Although it was based on animals, so it wasn't completely accurate. And he came up with hundreds of recipes for medicines, using ingredients that actually have an effect on the body, like opium, senna, castor oil and um ... ground-up lizards. Okay, that last one probably didn't have a *good* effect on the body –'

'Hey, listen to this!' said Rosy. 'Here's a quote from Galen about how great his medicines were: "All who drink of this medicine recover in a short time, except those whom it does not help, who all die. It is obvious, therefore, that it fails only in incurable cases."'

She glanced at Jaz and they suddenly found themselves doubled over with laughter.

'But seriously,' spluttered Rosy, some time later, 'it's a wonder Galen managed to fit through doorways, his head was so big. Look, here he is, calling all the other Roman doctors "dimwits".'

'Well, he must have been convincing,' said Jaz, 'because it says his work dominated medicine for the next thousand years. Where's my pen got to? I'd better make a note of – Look at the time! It's after four o'clock!

Dad will be wondering where I am!' She leaned over the desk and looked down at the front lawn, where her father was gathering up his shovels. 'I've got to go,' she said, snatching up her notebook and pen. 'I'll write up a summary of all this and bring it in tomorrow. You make sure you enlarge that photo of the little medieval painting so we can read the writing –'

She was out the door now, issuing orders over her shoulder from halfway down the corridor.

'*So* bossy,' Rosy said to the gargoyle. 'She's definitely choleric.'

The gargoyle gave her a phlegmatic smile.

Much, much later, Rosy lay in bed, gazing at the shadows cast upon her ceiling by the towering gum tree outside her window and sleepily turning over the events of the day in her head. She felt overloaded on food, after the huge celebratory dinner of Thai takeaway she'd had with her mum. The celebration was on account of Alison being asked to join some very important government committee as an adviser. Rosy was a bit fuzzy on the details of this, partly because she'd been so distracted by the delicious stir-fried noodles and crunchy snow peas and sticky black rice with coconut cream, but mostly because Alison's explanation had been full of science, which automatically made Rosy's brain switch off.

Chapter Four

When asked how she'd spent her day, Rosy had told her mum that she'd started helping Jaz with a project. Which was totally true, and it wasn't Rosy's fault if Alison assumed it was a *school* project. It was best not to tell parents too much, Rosy had learned. It was for their own good, really. They tended to stress out over nothing, which was bad for their blood pressure – and at their age, they had to be careful about that sort of thing.

Rosy kicked off the sheet covering her legs and turned over her pillow in an attempt to find a cool spot for her head. She wondered what Galen would have said about her mum's temperament. Alison was definitely a perfectionist, which would make her melancholic ... although she could be bossy, too ... But wait, had Jaz said what *her* mother was? Actually, now Rosy thought about it, she realised Jaz hadn't mentioned her mother at all – not once, the entire day. Jaz's mum and dad must be divorced, Rosy decided. Maybe Jaz's mum had left them.

Rosy sighed and rolled over onto her stomach, wishing she'd chosen a room that had air conditioning. There wasn't a whisper of a breeze, even though she'd pushed open the window as far as it would go ...

She drifted off into a restless sleep and dreamed that an ancient Egyptian mummy was shuffling through her room.

'Go away,' Rosy mumbled. She heard its unravelling bandages, as dry as paper, rustling to the floor, heard the scritch-scratch of its toenails against the floorboards. 'Stop that ...'

Then she fell into a much deeper sleep, and if there were more dreams, she didn't remember them. It wasn't until she was woken by a hot band of sunlight sliding across her room that Rosy saw what the mummy had done. Rosy looked at her desk and the floor below it, and she gasped.

CHAPTER FIVE

'The deepest sin against the human mind is to believe things without evidence.'
  ~ Attributed to T. H. Huxley

'Jaz,' Rosy hissed out of her window. 'Jaz! Up here! Quick!'

Jaz stopped on the gravel path that led from the car park and tilted her face up. 'What?' she said. She was carrying two bulging shopping bags and had her notebook tucked under one arm.

'You'll never guess – Oh, hang on, I'll come down!'

Rosy dashed out of her room, slamming the door behind her, and flew down the three flights of stairs to the foyer, where she almost collided with Jaz and her bags.

'Books,' said Jaz, before Rosy could ask. 'I went to the library last night and borrowed all I could find about the history of medicine.'

Rosy blinked at the bags, momentarily distracted. 'Your library lets you take out fifty books at a time?'

'I may have used some of my cousins' library cards as well. They won't notice. Here, can you look after the bags? I have to get the key to the Crypt for my dad.'

'Yes, well, hurry up!' Rosy shifted from foot to foot. 'Because something very weird has happened and you need to see it!'

She'd lost interest in the Crypt after Lynette had explained it was merely the room under the chapel where they stored old furniture – there were no mouldering tombs, no fluttering bats, not even any interesting-looking cobwebs, according to Lynette. After an excruciatingly long wait of at least five minutes, Jaz returned and Rosy was able to drag her upstairs. But Rosy came to a halt just outside her door.

'It's probably safe now,' she said, letting the bag of books she'd been carrying slump to the floor, 'although it's only fair to warn you first. You see, I've discovered that this room is ... HAUNTED.'

'Right,' said Jaz.

'Did you hear what I just said?'

'Can you please open the door?' said Jaz. 'This bag weighs a tonne.'

'You don't believe me,' said Rosy, planting her hands on her hips. 'Fine. Don't blame me if you faint from terror and hit your head on the floor and end up needing emergency brain surgery.'

She shoved open the door and marched inside. Jaz followed, arranged both bags of books neatly at the foot of the bed, then gazed slowly around the room – far too slowly for Rosy, who flung an arm in the direction of her desk.

'Over there!' she cried. 'Look what it did to my papers! They're in a complete mess!'

Chapter Five

'How can you tell?' asked Jaz, with a glance at Rosy's unmade bed and the pyjamas lying in a crumpled heap on the floor.

'Excuse me, I remember *exactly* where everything was on that desk last night and I'm telling you, those papers have been moved around! I was doing some sketches from memory of that Egyptian coffin and I left the paper right in the middle of the desk, in front of where I was sitting. But when I woke up this morning, it was over there, pushed right to the edge of the desk. And that's not all! You accidentally left your Eye of Horus photo behind yesterday and I found it *thrown in the bin.*'

She gave Jaz a significant look. With eyebrows and everything. Jaz remained blank-faced.

'Don't you understand?' said Rosy. '*That's* what it was after! It wanted the Eye of Horus. Its *own* Eye of Horus, snatched from its bandages as it lay in its coffin!'

'It?' said Jaz. 'You mean ... your ghost?'

'Ghost, mummy, same thing,' said Rosy, and she explained about her dream. 'What if there was a curse on whoever removed that Eye of Horus from the mummy? What if the mummy has been searching for its missing amulet for thousands of years? What if it suddenly realised that its Eye of Horus was *in this very building?*'

'What if I told you that you'd been watching too many scary movies?' said Jaz, crossing her arms over her chest. 'We don't even know if Dr Huxley's amulet *came* from a mummy. It could have been an ordinary

~ 63 ~

Egyptian necklace. And even if there *was* a mummy looking for its Eye of Horus and it somehow managed to travel all the way from ancient Egypt –'

'Or from the Nicholson Museum,' said Rosy. 'It could have been that boy, Horus. He could have overheard us talking yesterday.'

'– then wouldn't this *hypothetical* mummy have gone straight to the Senior Common Room, where the amulet actually *is*?'

'It came here first, looking for clues,' said Rosy. 'But hey, you're right! We'd better go and see if that cabinet's been smashed open!'

Jaz sighed. 'Did you have the window open last night?'

'Of course I did,' said Rosy. 'It was sweltering.'

'Well, there you go. A breeze blew in, rearranged the papers and happened to sweep one of them into the bin.'

'There wasn't any breeze. I told you, I just about melted into a puddle, it was so hot last night. Was there any breeze where you were?'

'No …' For the first time, Jaz appeared uncertain. She gazed at the desk, then at the bin. Then she shook her head vigorously. 'No, you're being as superstitious as the ancient Egyptians! There has to be a logical, rational explanation for this.'

'Like what?' Rosy threw both arms wide. 'Some person sneaking in here and searching through my papers while I was asleep? Mum wouldn't bother to do it secretly. She'd barge in and tell me to tidy up my

Chapter Five

room. There's no one else living in this building in the holidays. And how could anyone get into this room from outside? They'd have to be the world's skinniest person to fit through that window, and even then, how could they climb all the way up that stone wall? Unless they jumped from that overhanging tree branch ... but no, the branch would snap in two as soon as anyone tried to climb onto it. And my door was still locked when I got up. Although I guess there could be a spare key somewhere ...'

'There'd be one in the office,' said Jaz, frowning. 'What, you think it could've been Ms Boydell? You think she's guessed that we lost Dr Huxley's notes? And now she's looking for evidence?'

'Who's Ms Boydell?'

'Ms Susan Boydell. The bursar? The one who looks after the college finances?'

'Oh, you mean Lego Lady,' said Rosy. 'So that's what a bursar is. I thought it was an acronym. You know, BIG UNTIDY ROOM STOCKED WITH AUTHORISED RESOURCES, or something like that.'

'That would be BURSWAR,' said Jaz. 'And anyway –'

But Rosy had spotted something beneath the desk. 'A clue!' she cried, pouncing on it. She held it up between her finger and thumb. It was a fat yellow pellet. 'This could be *highly significant*.'

'I don't think so,' said Jaz. 'Those things ended up everywhere. I found one on the floor of Dad's ute this morning. It probably got squashed into my shoe and then fell off when I climbed in the ute.'

'Okay, scrap the significance.' Rosy tossed the pellet in the bin. 'But what about my mysterious visitor?'

'We can figure that out later,' said Jaz impatiently. 'We've got more important things to worry about right now. Remember, we're working to a deadline! And if it really *was* Ms Boydell, that's even more reason for us to focus on this. If we do a brilliant job, she won't be able to complain about us, will she? Here, have a look at these.'

Jaz pushed some sheets of paper into Rosy's hands, then busied herself unpacking her library books and sorting them into little piles on the desk. Rosy sat down on her bed and read the papers, which turned out to contain a long and extremely boring account of their research to date. But, as detailed as it was, it seemed to have left out some of the most important facts. Where, for example, were the mouse-munching Egyptian toddlers and the epileptic Roman vampires?

'Is it all right?' Jaz asked anxiously. 'I double-checked the dates in this book, *A Complete History of Medicine*. I wanted to type it all out, but my cousin was using the computer.'

'Mmm,' said Rosy. 'Yes, it's very ... thorough. I'll type it up later in a nice font and print it out.' She made a mental note to do a bit of rewriting as she typed. Double-checked dates were all very well, but she didn't want people reading it to fall into a tedium-induced coma. 'Okay.' She set the papers aside. 'So, what's next?'

'Did you enlarge the photo of that medieval religious painting so we could read the writing?'

Chapter Five

'Oh. Um …'

'Rosy!'

'Well, I was planning to do it this morning before breakfast, but then I had a few distractions. Like, you know, an ancient Egyptian mummy ransacking my room! Okay, fine, I'm doing it now. When Methuselah eventually wakes up … Hey, while we're waiting, go and check the Senior Common Room. See if the amulet's still there.'

Jaz huffed a bit, but went off, returning five minutes later to report that the door had been open because Ferdinand was vacuuming in there and that, as far as Jaz could tell, the cabinet and its contents were undisturbed.

'For the moment,' said Rosy ominously.

Jaz ignored this. 'Have you worked out what the writing says?' she asked, pulling a chair up to the desk.

'Unfortunately, the bigger I make the photo, the fuzzier it gets,' said Rosy. 'What do you think this letter is, a V or a U?'

'The first letter's definitely a V,' said Jaz, after a moment's scrutiny. 'But that letter there … it should be a vowel, shouldn't it, if it's a real word?'

'Could be an acronym,' suggested Rosy. 'Very Important Talisman Vitally …'

'No, it's a U,' Jaz decided.

'Vitus, then,' said Rosy. 'Was there a St Vitus? Let's see … Yes, St Vitus is the patron saint of comedians, dogs, dancers and young people. I like him already.'

'So our third object is a painting of St Vitus.' Jaz made a note of this. 'What else does it say about him?'

'Not much. Legend says he was martyred by the Roman Emperor Diocletian in about AD 303.'

'What does it mean by "martyred"?'

'Well, usually it means being killed in some really horrible way because the person refused to stop being a Christian. Wait, here's a website about Catholic saints. Wow, there are thousands of them! St Valentine, St Vigor, St Vincent ... St Vitus. Ah. You know how we thought our saint was standing in a pot of dirt?'

'He was buried alive?' said Jaz.

'No, he was boiled in a cauldron of molten lead. That was after they threw him into a den with a ravenous lion, except the lion just licked him in a friendly way. Hey, look, the cauldron in our painting has little lion paws for feet! I just noticed that. Cool. Yes, so the early Christians in Rome and Sicily built churches in honour of St Vitus. Then some of his relics – I guess that means his bones – were sent to France and Germany in the Middle Ages. He was declared one of the Fourteen Holy Helpers and was believed to have special healing powers, especially for those suffering from Sydenham's chorea, whatever that is.'

'That's actually pronounced kor-E-a,' said Jaz. 'It's where someone's muscles jerk uncontrollably.'

'How do you *know* all these things? It says here it's also called St Vitus's Dance. Wait, that sounds familiar ... Oh, of course! Dancing mania! That drawing by Bruegel!' Rosy's fingers flew over the keyboard. 'There, look, *The Epileptic Women of Molenbeek*!'

Jaz and Rosy studied the sketch of a procession of Flemish peasants. The men were either playing

Chapter Five

musical instruments or holding up the women, who were twisted into odd postures.

'They don't really have epilepsy,' Rosy explained. 'It's dancing mania. Dad told me about it. In Europe in the Middle Ages, there were these epidemics of compulsive dancing, where crowds of people would dance till they dropped. They couldn't stop themselves. It would go on for days, or even weeks, and some of them actually died from heart attacks and exhaustion and stuff. And look, it says that in Strasbourg one year, they danced into a chapel where they saw a picture of St Vitus and they all fell down and worshipped him and were cured. It was a miracle!'

'It was *not* a miracle,' said Jaz, who'd also been reading the article that accompanied the drawing. 'Because they weren't sick. They were uneducated peasants in a world ruled by the Catholic Church, and every now and then, they'd throw themselves into a religious frenzy. It says here they used to report seeing visions of the Virgin Mary while they danced. And when musicians started accompanying them, it only encouraged more people to join in. It's not as though there was much other entertainment in those days.'

'It *could* have been a disease, though,' said Rosy. 'Some of them might have had that chorea thing, if it makes people's arms and legs jerk about. And it says *here* that some episodes of dancing mania could have been due to ergotism, also known as St Anthony's Fire, which is, um ... Oh, a fungus that grows on rye causes it. The fungus is chemically related to a drug called LSD and it causes hallucinations and seizures. In other words – dancing mania! Oh, except it also caused terrible burning sensations and gangrene, which made people's hands and feet drop off. I guess that would make dancing a bit difficult.'

'And then I suppose they prayed to St Anthony for a cure,' scoffed Jaz.

'Well, what else could they do? It was probably more helpful than bloodletting. Look at this statue of St Anthony. He's got such a kind, calm face. He's not even bothered by all the flames crawling up his legs – What are you doing?'

Jaz was scrabbling through her piles of books. 'You reminded me of something ... Oh, here it is. I started reading this last night. It's about the Black Death.'

'Just a bit of light bedtime reading, then?'

'It *was* pretty depressing,' Jaz admitted. 'Did you know that the Black Death killed more than twenty million people in only three years? Twenty million! That's almost the entire population of Australia. In some parts of France and Spain, three out of every four people died. Can you imagine?'

'This was the plague, right?'

'Yes, but there were a few outbreaks of plague in the Middle Ages,' said Jaz, flipping through the pages. 'Let's see, the first started in the sixth century – the Plague of Justinian. That killed about half the population of Europe. Then it started again in China about eight hundred years later. It reached Constantinople in 1347 and had spread all through the Middle East and Europe by 1350.'

'It was carried by rats, wasn't it?' said Rosy. 'Rats on ships. I remember, we did this at school.'

'Well, it was really caused by bacteria called *Yersinia pestis* that live inside fleas. The fleas travelled on the rats, the rats got sick and died, then the fleas jumped onto humans and infected them as well. That's the hypothesis, anyway, and there's lots of evidence for it when you look at the historical descriptions of the Black Death. Scientists have even dug up skeletons from plague graves and found *Yersinia pestis* DNA in the skeletons' teeth. But the bacteria caused a few different forms of plague. With pneumonic plague, you coughed up blood and died within a few days, but first you'd infect anyone you'd sneezed or coughed on. With bubonic plague, you'd live a bit longer but you'd vomit up blood, have seizures and develop lumps in your neck, armpits and groin, which would ooze –'

'Thanks, I think that's enough detail,' said Rosy.

'Of course, they didn't know about bacteria back then,' said Jaz. 'Some people thought it was due to the position of the planets causing bad air, but most people believed the Church when it said that this was God's punishment. So bands of flagellants would wander around the country. They were people who whipped themselves to atone for their sins. They spread panic – and probably spread the disease as well.

'Then the Pope declared that the River Rhône was sacred, so people threw dead victims into the river instead of burying them – that's the same water they used for washing and drinking, of course. People fasted, they prayed, they went on barefooted pilgrimages, they bought holy relics – oh, and by the way, it says here that relics weren't just bones of martyred saints. A relic could be a saint's glove or rosary beads, or just a vial of oil that had *touched* something that supposedly belonged to a saint. People paid a fortune for holy cures, none of which actually worked. Then they started blaming the Jews, saying that Jews had poisoned the air or the water. There were all these massacres in Germany, where thousands of Jews were burnt alive and whole communities were wiped out.'

'That's so horrible!'

'I know,' said Jaz. 'But it's weird, isn't it, how superstitious people were? It's like Europe went *backwards* during the Middle Ages. In ancient Greece, you had Aristotle talking about observation and facts and finding evidence to back up theories. Even Galen based a lot of his ideas on experiments. But once Christianity got going, people stopped *thinking*.'

'Well, that's because they were all busy dying of plague. If half of your town suddenly dropped dead, I bet *you'd* have problems thinking rationally, too.'

'Maybe that's why Dr Huxley had a painting of St Vitus in his collection?' mused Jaz. 'To show how religion affected the history of medicine …'

'But there must have been some doctors around then.'

'Yes, there's a bit about them in this next chapter, except their ideas weren't much better. They used to cut open live frogs and pigeons and stick them on the plague sores to draw out the poison. And there was bloodletting, of course.'

Chapter Five

'Of course,' said Rosy. 'Great idea! Why not splash around some plague-infected blood? And what on Earth is *that*?' She pointed at a bizarre illustration in the book.

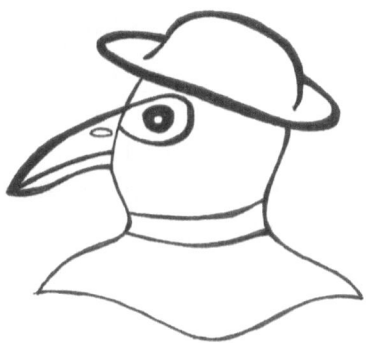

'A plague doctor,' read out Jaz. 'They wore long coats made of leather, a brimmed hat and a mask with glass eyeholes and a long beak. The beak was filled with dried roses, cloves, camphor or a sponge soaked in vinegar, which was supposed to protect the plague doctor from bad air. He also carried a long white cane so he could examine patients without touching them.'

'Look, it says Nostradamus was a plague doctor,' said Rosy. 'The same Nostradamus who made all those weird prophecies!'

'Well, he did have some sensible advice about the plague,' said Jaz. 'He was against bloodletting and he recommended fresh air, clean water and proper disposal of dead bodies.' She turned the page. 'Oh, look, this is interesting. The plague doctor's job wasn't just to care for plague victims, but also to record the number of deaths and look for a cure. It was the first time cities really started to think about public health. For instance, in 1377, Ragusa, a Venetian colony, decided to isolate ships for forty days after they arrived, to make sure sailors and cargo were truly free of the plague before they left the ship. That's why it's called quarantine now, because *quarantina* is Italian for "forty days". And in Milan ... Oh. When the plague reached Milan, authorities bricked up the doors and windows of the three affected households, sealing all the people and animals inside.'

Rosy stared at her, aghast. 'And they all died?'

'Yes, but the city was saved. Hardly anyone died of the plague in Milan that year, compared to other places. And the idea spread across Europe, so that by 1543, there were official plague rules in England. Plague-ridden houses had to mark the sign of the cross on their doors. People who'd been in contact with plague victims had to quarantine themselves or carry a white stick if they went out. Infected straw and clothes had to be burned and streets had to be kept clean. And most people seemed to have stopped believing it was caused by sinfulness – maybe because priests and nuns were dying of plague just as much as everyone else.'

'Wait, this plague was still going on in 1543? It lasted two hundred years?'

'It was a series of epidemics and it kept coming back in Europe until the eighteenth century. The last outbreak in England was the Great Plague of London in 1665.'

Chapter Five

'And then it just went away? I guess it must have, because no one gets plague now, do they?'

'I don't know,' said Jaz. 'This book only goes up to 1666.'

'I'd better check on that,' said Rosy, turning back to Methuselah. 'Let's see ... Oh no, it's still around! Some poor kid got bubonic plague a few years ago when she went camping in Colorado! And thousands of people still get pneumonic plague in Africa each year! And *millions* died of the plague in China and India about a hundred years ago. I'd never even heard about that, had you? It was called "The Third Pandemic". What's the difference between a pandemic and an epidemic?'

'A pandemic is bigger. It spreads over a whole continent or the whole world. So I guess the Black Death was really a pandemic, not an epidemic,' Jaz explained.

'Oh, okay. Hey, did you know there was an epidemic of bubonic plague here in Sydney, too? A series of epidemics, actually, between 1900 and 1925. About five hundred people died. And it was Australian scientists who helped prove that the plague was spread by fleas on rats. Here, write their names down. John Ashburton Thompson, Frank Tidswell and William Armstrong. Do you want me to spell any of those?'

Jaz shook her head. 'No, because they're not medieval. I think we've got a bit off the track here. Remember, we're meant to be researching the painting of St Vitus. I think Dr Huxley wanted it to represent the influence of religion on medicine in the Middle Ages.'

'So you don't want to look at this photo taken in 1900 of the City of Sydney Ratcatchers standing behind a huge pile of dead rats?'

'Not really.'

'No, I don't blame you. It's totally disgusting. Okay, what else is there to know about medicine and religion in the Middle Ages?'

'Well, I want to find out more about women healers.'

'Ooh, witches!'

'I was thinking of nuns,' said Jaz. 'In one of these books, they mentioned a nun called Hildegard who wrote a book about medicine.'

'Let's do witches first ... Methuselah? Methuselah, do you have something against witches? Or nuns? Or women?'

Methuselah's screen remained stubbornly blank.

Rosy sighed. 'I need a break, anyway. My brain's full. Hey, you want to come for a walk to the shop? Mum didn't have time to buy printer cartridges yesterday, but she's left me her staff discount card and some money. I want to take some photos of all those cool old buildings, too.'

CHAPTER SIX

'Formerly, when religion was strong and science weak, men mistook magic for medicine ...'
~ Thomas Szasz

Jaz went off to tell her dad about their shopping expedition and Rosy waited for her at the front of New College. Across the road was a little booth for the university security guard who answered visitors' questions and handed out maps and checked that cars had valid parking permits. As it was the middle of the summer holidays and there were hardly any cars around, and no lost or confused people, he was not exactly overwhelmed with work. At the moment, he was standing in the doorway of his booth, making a face at a squashed Coke can that was half-buried in the adjacent flowerbed.

Rosy was irresistibly reminded of Amelia Pinkerton, a prefect at her school, who'd once given Rosy and her friend a detention because they hadn't picked up a chip packet that someone else had dropped. As the guard pursed his lips and shook his head, a snort of laughter escaped Rosy's nose. The security guard whipped his head round at the sound, scowled, then marched across the road.

'Move along, please!' he snapped. 'It's an offence to obstruct a university footpath.'

Rosy looked at him – he was much younger than she'd first thought – and then down at her feet. She was sitting on the low stone wall with her toes dangling above the path. Could you obstruct something when you weren't actually *on* it? Even if she stuck her legs straight out, there'd still be plenty of room for people to walk past.

'*Now*, not next week,' insisted the guard. 'Pedestrians require unhindered access to the footpath.'

Rosy looked right, then left. The path was completely deserted. 'But ... there aren't any pedestrians,' she ventured.

'Loitering on university property is also an offence,' he said. 'Move –'

'She isn't *on* university property,' said Jaz, appearing out of nowhere. 'She's on the grounds of a private residential college, so it's none of your business what she does. She can sit wherever she likes!'

The guard gaped at her, momentarily speechless. Then he looked over her shoulder and his eyes widened. 'Is that your father?' he asked. Rosy turned and saw Jaz's dad single-handedly yanking a dead tree out of the garden. It was a fairly small tree. Still, he looked pretty intimidating – although not half as intimidating as Jaz, who was doing fierce eyebrows at the guard.

'I know you,' said the guard slowly, pointing his finger at her. 'You're Tej's little sister.'

Chapter Six

'No, I'm not,' said Jaz.

'Yes, you are,' he insisted. 'Tej! Tej Singh!'

'I'm *not* his sister,' said Jaz. 'He's my cousin.'

'You *know* this guy?' Rosy asked Jaz.

'His name's Mohammad and he was in the same year as my cousin at school,' said Jaz. 'He's only eighteen. He's not a proper security guard.'

'I am so!' cried Mohammad. 'I've got a uniform and a badge and everything!' Then he seemed to realise this didn't sound very authoritative and he straightened his spine and lifted his chin. 'Ahem! So if you have no further questions, I'll return to my duties now.'

Then he spun on one heel and marched back to his booth.

'Was he a prefect at your school?' Rosy asked Jaz, as they set off up the road.

'Vice Captain,' said Jaz. 'And Canteen Monitor.'

'I knew it,' said Rosy. 'Did he ever make you pick up chip packets?'

'What? No, he was just really annoying. Here, hold this.' She passed Rosy a water bottle and opened the book that she'd tucked under her arm.

'You can't read while you're walking,' protested Rosy.

'Yes, I can,' said Jaz. 'I do it all the time. I do it on the way to school each morning.'

'Don't you trip over and bump into things?'

'No. I know the footpath. And my cousin Kirin warns me if there's anything in the way.'

'Oh. Okay,' said Rosy. 'Well, I'll be your cousin for now.' She was feeling quite kindly towards Jaz, after

Jaz had rushed to her defence so ferociously. 'What's the book about?'

'Women healers in the Middle Ages.'

'Witches?'

'Wise women,' corrected Jaz. 'The old women in the villages who helped deliver babies and made herbal remedies.'

'Potions and lotions,' said Rosy, nodding. 'And magic spells.'

'Okay, some of them *did* use magical incantations and charms – but it's not as though doctors of the time were any better. It says here the physician to King Edward II had a doctorate in medicine from Oxford and *he* thought the best cure for a toothache was to write "In the name of the Father, the Son and the Holy Ghost, Amen" on the patient's jaw. Or else to touch a caterpillar with a needle, then hold the needle against the sore tooth.'

'At least he didn't recommend bloodletting,' said Rosy.

'He probably recommended that, as well,' said Jaz. 'Actually, doctors had made some progress in that area by then. They weren't just slicing open veins anymore. They'd started sucking blood out with leeches.'

'*You* might call leeches "progress",' said Rosy. 'I don't. But go on about women healers.'

'Well, apart from the village wise women, there were nuns who nursed the sick and wounded. For example, the Hôtel-Dieu, the oldest hospital in Paris, began as a hostel near St Christopher's Church, where the sisters washed, bandaged and fed the sick. When

Chapter Six

the Black Death arrived in 1348, the sisters refused to abandon their patients, even after all the university-trained doctors had fled and the patients were piled up six in a bed. And one of the most famous women in medieval medicine was Hildegard of Bingen. She was enclosed in a nunnery at the age of eight by her family, and went on to establish her own convent and write several books about healing.'

'Overhanging branch coming up on your right.'

'Thanks,' said Jaz, veering left without raising her eyes from the page. 'Two of Hildegard's books, *Physica* and *Causae et Curae,* described how different sorts of animals, plants, minerals and precious stones could be used in medicine. For instance, she wrote about a type of daisy called tansy: "Tansy is hot and a little damp and is good against all superfluous flowing humours and whoever suffers from catarrh and has a cough, let him eat tansy."'

'So she believed in all the ancient Greek stuff about humours?'

'And in astrology,' said Jaz. 'Oh, and unicorns. Her cure for leprosy included unicorn liver.'

Rosy looked up at the stone archway they were approaching. Among the fantastical creatures carved into the sandstone was a wild-eyed, rearing unicorn. Most of the unicorn's horn was missing. 'What about *horn* of unicorn?' Rosy said, nudging Jaz and pointing upwards. 'You reckon Hildegard's been here?'

'Her leprosy cure also contained lion heart,' noted Jaz. They shifted their gazes to the snarling lion on the other side of the archway. There was a jagged scar along his ribs, clumsily patched with mortar.

'No wonder he looks angry,' said Rosy. 'Shame on you, Hildegard! Ripping the hearts out of poor innocent lions! Especially as your cure didn't even work! Or did it?' She turned to Jaz.

'Of course it didn't work,' said Jaz. 'It used ingredients that didn't *exist*. She didn't even do any experiments, she just made up recipes in her head. Hang on – why are we outside the museum? I thought you said we were going to the shop?'

'We are. It's on the other side of the quadrangle. But as we're here, we *could* pop in and see if Horus the Boy Mummy is –'

'No,' said Jaz firmly.

'I guess he'd be back in his glass case now, anyway,' said Rosy. 'Pretending to be harmless. Hi, Naomi!' They waved at the museum guide, who was sitting at the reception desk with a cup of coffee and a thick book. She glanced up, smiled and waved back, and Rosy and Jaz walked on, out into the brightness of the quadrangle.

'So, returning to medieval women healers,' said Rosy. 'Didn't any of them become doctors? You said doctors were being trained in universities by then.'

'Yes, there's a bit about that here ... Sicily was the first place to require doctors to pass an exam and get a medical licence, and that was in 1140. Then other places in Europe started doing the same thing. But women weren't allowed to attend universities, so they

Chapter Six

couldn't qualify as doctors. And in France, doctors also had to take Church vows and women weren't allowed to do that either, so women really, *really* couldn't be doctors there.

'In 1322, there was a famous trial in Paris, where they charged a woman called Jacqueline Felicie with being an unlicensed physician. At least six witnesses testified at her trial, saying she'd cured them of diseases that licensed doctors hadn't been able to treat. She also refused to accept payment unless her patient got better, so it's not as though she was ripping people off. Plus, she pointed out that lots of women patients *preferred* to be examined by a woman doctor. But the court still found her guilty and made her pay a huge fine.'

'That is *so* unfair.'

'It gets worse. In 1486, a Catholic priest wrote *Malleus Maleficarum*, an official guide to witch-hunting. He said witches could cause any disease, "even leprosy or epilepsy", and that "no one does more harm to the Catholic Faith than midwives". He meant wise women. If a wise woman helped someone give birth and the baby died or was malformed, the wise woman must have sacrificed the child to the devil, so she must be punished. Oh, and he also said sickness was sent by God as a punishment for sins. So if prayers didn't cure the disease, but the wise woman's herbal remedies did, it must be because she was in league with the devil. Thousands of women across Europe were interrogated and killed in horrible ways, all thanks to this book.'

Rosy shook her head angrily.

'There was this English woman,' Jaz went on, as they climbed the steps to the shop, 'called Ursula Kemp. She cured her neighbour of lameness, but the neighbour refused to pay the fee and they quarrelled. So when the neighbour's lameness came back and her baby died, she accused Ursula of witchcraft. At the trial, Ursula's eight-year-old son claimed his mother had four familiars – a toad, a lamb and a couple of cats – which she fed with beer and cake and her own blood, then sent out at night to kill people. Ursula was tortured until she confessed, and she and several other women in the village were hanged in 1582.'

'I wish she really *had* been a witch,' said Rosy. 'She could have risen from the grave and wreaked her vengeance on all those cruel, stupid people. Sorry, not you,' she said to the woman behind the counter, who was looking askance at them. 'Can I please get one of those printer cartridges? And a colour one, too? Thanks. Hey, Jaz, this cream paper's nice, isn't it? Like parchment. We could print out the final draft of our research on that. You think? I've got enough money.'

'Uh-huh,' said Jaz, still engrossed in her book. 'There were also the Witches of Warboys in 1593 ...'

A student loomed beside them at the counter, juggling a steaming cup of takeaway coffee, a mobile phone and a couple of bulky folders.

'Hi, Marcus,' said Rosy. Today his T-shirt read, 'MICROBIOLOGIST: WILL WORK FOR ICE-CREAM'.

'Oh, look, it's the detectives,' he said. 'Solved your mystery yet?'

Chapter Six

'Our investigation is progressing satisfactorily,' Rosy said, holding his coffee cup for him as he paid for a travel card.

'Good to hear,' he said, retrieving the cup. 'Thanks. Well, back to the grindstone. See you later, Monsieur Poirot and Miss Marple.' He waved his free elbow at them and loped out again.

'Agatha Christie,' Rosy explained to Jaz, who was looking confused. 'Obviously, I'm Monsieur Poirot because I can speak French. That makes you Miss Marple. You may look like a sweet little old lady, but you have a mind like a steel trap.'

They went back outside.

'So, anyway,' Rosy continued, 'was it just women who were persecuted as witches?'

'Mostly women,' said Jaz. 'They were supposed to be more susceptible to the devil.'

'That's so sexist,' said Rosy. 'I mean, what about Faust?' She gestured at the fountain across the road.

'Who?'

'You know, the story about Dr Faust? And his deal with the devil? That stone head over there is supposed to be Mephistopheles. Dad told me it was based on a design by Norman Lindsay, so you'd think the university would take better care of it, 'cause he's a really famous Australian artist, isn't he? Look, its poor nose has fallen right off.'

'I have no idea what you're talking about,' said Jaz. 'You mean, that thing that looks like Voldemort, spitting water into the pool?'

'Well, Mephistopheles *was* sort of like Voldemort. There was this doctor, see, Dr Faust, and he wanted to know everything. Then Mephistopheles turned up and said the devil would give Faust unlimited knowledge, but in return, Faust had to give his soul to the devil. So Faust said, "Okay. Why not?" and he got everything he'd ever wanted in life, and then a few years later, the devil said, "Right, that's enough life for you. Now I get your soul for eternity." And Faust died and went to hell. And you know the spookiest bit?'

'What?'

'There really *was* a Dr Faust. He was a magician and alchemist in Germany, and the Church reckoned he'd done a deal with the devil. He died in a big explosion while he was doing an experiment and all that was left behind were his eyeballs.'

'Riiight.'

'It's true. You can look it up! Dr Faust. Or maybe Dr Faustus. Something like that.'

Jaz continued to look sceptical. 'And he was an actual *alchemist*,' she said. 'What, you mean turning lead into gold – that sort of thing?'

'Yes, and finding the Elixir of Life, which cured all diseases and made you immortal if you drank enough of it.'

'As if that's even *possible*.'

'Anything is possible,' said Rosy.

Jaz slammed her book shut, in order to concentrate on arguing, then looked around, frowning. 'Wait, isn't that the sports field over there? We could have taken a

Chapter Six

short cut across it to get to the shop. We didn't need to go all that way past the museum!'

'We took the scenic route,' said Rosy serenely.

When they got back to New College, they discovered Ferdinand was polishing all the refectory tables, so they took their lunch out to a shady bench in the front garden. Jaz had brought down some of her library books from Rosy's room, because she wanted to find out more about alchemy.

'There's no mention of a Dr Faust in this index,' she said to Rosy. '*Or* Faustus. There's a lot about Paracelsus, though. He's supposed to have been the most famous alchemist of his time.'

'Was he German? No, he couldn't be – Paracelsus doesn't sound like a German name.'

'Actually, he was born in Switzerland in about 1493 and was named Theophrastus Philippus Aureolus Bombastus von Hohenheim. But he called himself Paracelsus –'

'Because it was easier to spell.'

'– because he believed he was greater than Celsus. Remember Celsus, that Roman doctor who identified the four signs of inflammation and wrote all those medical texts?'

'So Paracelsus had an ego almost as big as Galen's,' said Rosy.

'No, even bigger. Here's a Paracelsus quote: "Let me tell you this: every little hair on my neck knows more than you and all your scribes, and my shoe buckles are more learned than your Galen and Avicenna, and my beard has more experience than all your high colleges."'

'Shoe buckles!' crowed Rosy. 'Take that, Galen! But did Paracelsus actually do anything useful?'

'Well, he was one of the first to use chemistry in medicine, because he thought diseases were due to an imbalance of minerals in the body. Although he *also* claimed that poisons falling from the stars caused this, so a lot of his cures involved astrological charms. He came up with the idea that "the dose makes the poison", which meant a chemical might be helpful in tiny doses, but dangerous in large doses. What else ...' Jaz flipped through the pages. 'Oh, he invented a miracle cure he called "laudanum", which was basically opium dissolved in alcohol, so it was a pretty effective painkiller. He wrote lots of books about medicine and surgery. But I think he mostly just went around annoying other doctors. It says here he held a public ceremony to burn a whole lot of traditional medical books by Galen and Avicenna.'

'Who's Avicenna? I don't think we've come across him before, have we?'

Jaz consulted the index. 'Here he is. Avicenna was –'

'Better known as Abu 'Ali al-Husayn ibn 'Abd Allah ibn Sina!'

They turned around to see Mohammad's head sticking up over the top of the college wall.

'Also known as the Father of Medicine,' he went on, 'as well as –'

'No, he wasn't,' said Rosy. 'That was Hippocrates.'

Chapter Six

'Shouldn't you be in your *booth*?' Jaz said to Mohammad, but he simply moved along to a lower part of the wall, in order to lean over it more comfortably.

'– as well as one of the greatest thinkers and scientists of all time,' Mohammad continued loudly. 'Because while the Western world was stuck in the Dark Ages, the Father of *Modern* Medicine was writing his fourteen-volume encyclopaedia, describing all the diseases of the time, what caused them, how to treat them, how to test a new medicine, as well as plenty of good advice about exercise, diet, massage and sleep. And of course, before him had been the great Muhammad ibn Zakariya al-Razi, who wrote dozens of books about anatomy, surgery and diseases. And before *that* was 'Ali ibn Rabban al-Tabari's medical compendium. If not for the great scholars of the Islamic Golden Age, who managed to preserve and translate all the ancient wisdom of Greece and Rome –'

'Okay. Thanks,' said Jaz. 'You can go now.'

'– there would *be* no medicine! Not without the Persians! Even that word, *alchemy*. Where do you think it comes from, eh? Arabic! *Al-kīmiyā*. Who do you think first worked out how to filter and distil and crystallise? Who first described how to make syrups, elixirs, pure essences? Who set up the first apothecary shops?'

'Why are you still here?' said Jaz.

'It is a *little* bit interesting,' Rosy conceded.

'Well, *I* could have told you all that about Avicenna,' snapped Jaz. 'I bet it's all in this book! And who would

Dr Huxley's Bequest

you rather believe, the doctor who wrote this book or some random trainee parking inspector?'

'Soon to be studying *medicine* at this prestigious university,' said Mohammad over one shoulder, as he sauntered off.

'What!' said Jaz, but he'd disappeared. 'Him!' she said to Rosy. '*Medicine*!'

'Guess he must be pretty smart, then.'

'I can't believe he's applied to study *medicine*,' fumed Jaz. 'Here! Anyway, the exam results aren't even out yet. He doesn't even know if he got accepted.'

'Still,' said Rosy.

'He'd make a *terrible* doctor,' said Jaz. 'He's such an annoying know-it-all.'

Rosy maintained a tactful silence.

CHAPTER SEVEN

'Good science and good art both require imagination.'
~ Jenny Pollak

'He looks quite cheerful, doesn't he?' said Rosy. 'Considering he's dead.'

Having finished lunch and their investigation into medieval medicine, Rosy and Jaz had returned to Rosy's room, where they were currently examining their photo of Dr Huxley's next object.

'Although I suppose skeletons always *do* look like they're grinning,' Rosy added. 'On account of not having any lips.'

The skeleton in the framed picture was arranged in a casual upright pose, one leg crossed over the other, one elbow propped on a tomb, the curled back of the skeleton's hand supporting its skull. It was contemplating a second, disembodied skull, which was on the verge of rolling off the lid of the tomb.

'And notice they're all on the edge of a cliff,' said Rosy. 'Symbolic, that is.'

Meanwhile, Jaz was trying to decipher the writing along the top of the page. 'Even if it weren't in Latin, it'd be impossible to figure out,' she complained. 'They *still* haven't learned that V and U aren't meant to look the same. And the words are all different sizes and fonts and that skull's drawn right in the middle of the text!'

'I'll copy it out exactly as it's printed, then we can have a think about it.' Rosy turned to a fresh page of Jaz's notebook and wrote:

> 164 ANDREÆ VESALII BRVXELLENSIS
> **HVMANI COR- PORIS OSSIVM CÆ**
> *TERIS QVASSV- STINENT PARTIBVS*
> LIBERORVM, SVAQVE SEDE POSITORVM EX
> *latere delineatio.*

There was also an inscription on the tomb, which said,

> VIVITVR IN-
> GENIO,
> CÆTERA MOR-
> TIS ERVNT.

They stared at this for a while.

'I think the first line is either the title of the book or the author's name,' said Jaz, 'assuming "164" is a page number.'

'And the different fonts and sizes are probably just because the printer got bored and wanted to mix things up a bit.'

'And every syllable needs a vowel,' said Jaz. 'And a Q usually has a U after it. It does in English, anyway.'

'And I think "ossium" means "bones",' said Rosy. 'Because an ossuary is a room where they store the bones of dead people. And "mortis" must have

Chapter Seven

something to do with death, because a mortician is an undertaker and a mortuary is a – What?'

'Nothing.'

'You were giving me a funny look.'

'They're odd words for you to know, that's all.'

'I know heaps of words,' said Rosy. 'That's what my English teacher said in my report: "Rosy has an extensive vocabulary." Or maybe it was "exhaustive". Or "exhausting". Dad said it meant I talked too much in class. But anyway, I don't think it's weird to know about ossuaries! Lots of old churches have them. There are chapels in Europe *made* of bones. It's symbolic, isn't it? Of how, no matter who we are, we all end up as a pile of bones. I think that's very profound. And by the way, in French, you say "Bruxelles" instead of Brussels, so I think this book must be from there.'

And when they typed 'Andreae Vesalii Bruxellensis' into Methuselah's search engine, he promptly informed them that a famous anatomist called Andreas Vesalius had indeed been born in Brussels in 1514.

'Ha!' said Rosy.

'The author of one of the most influential books ever written on human anatomy, *De Humani Corporis Fabrica*,' read out Jaz. 'Which means "On the Fabric of the Human Body". So I guess "humani corporis ossium" means "the bones of the human body".'

Methuselah proved surprisingly helpful at translating the rest of the Latin.

'That's because Latin is Methuselah's first language,' Rosy said. 'That's what they all spoke a thousand years ago, when he was made.'

'So,' said Jaz, 'the tomb says something like "Intelligence lives, the rest eventually dies" or "Genius is life, the rest will belong to death".'

'Very profound.' Rosy nodded.

'And the other sentence is something along the lines of: "Drawings of the bones of the human body, supported freely and seen from the side".'

'Slightly less profound,' said Rosy. 'Hey – look at this! A university scanned all the illustrations from *De Humani Corporis Fabrica* and put them up online. And they're ... um ... they're ... Wow.'

There were dozens of exquisitely detailed drawings of a man, in various lifelike poses, being systematically stripped of his skin, his muscles, his sinews, all his internal organs, until he was nothing but a bare skeleton leaning against a tomb. The title page of the book showed a doctor slicing open a corpse on the stage of an ornate theatre, surrounded by dozens of interested observers, including two cherubs, a dog and a monkey.

'Well ... I guess they'd stopped disapproving of human dissection by 1543,' said Jaz faintly.

'It looks like they'd started selling tickets to the general public,' said Rosy. 'Although those spectators *could* all be medical students, I suppose. Okay, maybe not the dog ...'

Jaz was scrolling down the page. 'I think they *are* meant to be medical students. Because it says here that Andreas Vesalius was a lecturer in surgery and anatomy, and that dissections of human bodies had been going on at European universities since at least

Chapter Seven

1318. The Church didn't actually forbid it, as long as the body was given a Christian burial afterwards. *De Humani Corporis Fabrica* wasn't the first anatomy book to be published, though – just the most successful. Apparently Vesalius was really skilful with a knife, as well as knowing off by heart all the classical medical texts written by –'

Rosy pulled a face. 'Oh, not Galen.'

'Yes, but Vesalius wasn't afraid to argue if he found evidence that the textbooks were wrong. Galen said there were holes in the middle of the heart so that blood could flow from one side to the other. But Vesalius couldn't find any of those holes and he said so. And he contradicted Galen about the shape of the liver and about how many bones made up the jawbone and breastbone. Of course, Galen's ideas came from cutting up apes, not humans, and Vesalius pointed that out, too.'

'Go, Vesalius!'

'But then all the Galen supporters started attacking Vesalius. They said Galen *had* studied human bodies. They said if there were any mistakes in the textbooks, it must be because Galen's manuscripts had been translated wrongly. Oh, and here's the best one – they said that any differences Vesalius found were because human bodies in 1543 weren't as pure and perfect as ancient Roman bodies.' Jaz raised an eyebrow.

'Ha! As if.'

'Vesalius did make mistakes of his own, but he fixed some of them in his revised edition. He didn't mind admitting he'd been wrong. He *encouraged* his students to check his work, and their own. He said you had to observe things yourself to discover the truth. That's *science*, that is.' And Jaz gave a nod of approval.

'But it's art, too,' said Rosy, who'd scrolled back to a portrait of a man caught mid-stride in a country lane, his face tilted towards the sun, each muscle and sinew of his flayed body carefully outlined and shaded. 'I mean, these muscle men are a bit ... well, disturbing, but that's only because they're so *vivid*. Look at how carefully the artist sketched the background, with the road winding away through the countryside to the village. Look at this tiny lizard climbing the rocks near the skeleton's feet. It's like Vesalius wanted to show that these were real people who'd only just stopped being alive. They're not pieces of meat on a slab – they're human beings. Did he do all these drawings himself?'

They both studied Methuselah's screen. 'It looks like no one knows for sure,' said Jaz at last. 'It could've been him, because he illustrated an earlier book about anatomy. But it could have been an artist called Jan Stephan van Calcar or it could have been a whole lot of different artists from the studio of um, Titian?'

'Oh, *Titian*,' repeated Rosy – pronouncing it Tee-shan – as though Jaz had mentioned an old friend. 'Yeah, he's great.' She settled back in her chair. 'And you know, Leonardo da Vinci did some awesome anatomical drawings around this time, too. And I just remembered – there's a painting by Rembrandt called *The Anatomy Lesson*.'

'Was that at the same time as Vesalius?'

'No, a bit later, in the 1600s. It has a doctor pointing out muscles on a dead body to all these other doctors and there's a big anatomy book propped up in the corner – hey, that's probably *De Humani Corporis Fabrica*! And – Oh!' Rosy clapped her hands in excitement. 'Michelangelo's hidden brain anatomy! You know the Sistine Chapel?'

'No.'

'Yes, you do. It's a chapel in the Vatican and Michelangelo painted its ceiling with scenes from the Bible. There's an incredibly famous panel called *Creation of Adam*, where God's floating in the sky supported by a bunch of angels, and he's stretching down his finger, and Adam's lying naked on the earth, reaching up with *his* hand, and their fingers are nearly, nearly touching –'

'Oh, yes. With God in a cloud.'

'Actually, he's surrounded by a billowing red cloak.' Rosy was typing into Methuselah's search engine as she spoke. 'And guess what? It's shaped exactly like a human brain, seen from the side. *Exactly.*' She swivelled the screen around to face Jaz. 'See? All the blood vessels and nerves and folds and bumps of the brain match up perfectly with the outlines of the cloak and the angels' legs and that trailing green scarf.'

'That's ... pretty impressive,' Jaz admitted, after prolonged scrutiny. 'But how could Michelangelo know so much about brain anatomy? He couldn't have looked it up in *De Humani Corporis Fabrica*, because he painted this two years before Vesalius was born.'

'Well, Michelangelo was a genius, wasn't he? Like Leonardo. And look, it says here that Michelangelo started dissecting dead bodies when he was still a teenager. That's how he could do all those amazingly realistic sculptures and drawings and paintings of the human body. Oh, and by the way, it's not just *Creation of Adam* that has hidden anatomy in it. Here's the first panel from the Sistine Chapel, *Separation of Light from Darkness*, and see, there's another brain hidden in God's neck.'

'Oh, yes,' said Jaz, tilting her head for a better perspective. 'The brainstem, from below.'

'I like *Creation of Adam* best, though,' said Rosy. 'It's like God is handing over intelligence to the first human.'

'Or Michelangelo is saying that God only exists inside human brains.'

'No, I don't think so. The Pope wouldn't have been very happy if he'd found a big atheist message painted right across the middle of his chapel. More likely, Michelangelo was saying God was super smart.'

'Well, Michelangelo was certainly smart,' said Jaz. 'Teaching himself all that about anatomy.'

'He was a *genius*. I said that. But hey, I wonder where all those anatomists got their dead bodies from? Vesalius must have gone through dozens of bodies when he was working on his book. It's not like they had fridges back then – he couldn't just keep using the same body.'

'I think they mostly used executed criminals,' Jaz said. 'That article about Vesalius said he once cut down

Chapter Seven

a man hanging from a roadside gallows and took the body home to turn it into a skeleton. And his students stole at least one body from a grave.'

'Body-snatchers!' said Rosy. 'Ooh, that reminds me of Burke and ... Hare? I think that's what they were called. This was in Edinburgh in the 1800s, when there were all these body-snatchers around, robbing fresh graves and selling the bodies to medical schools for dissection practice. I guess they weren't executing as many criminals by then.'

'They were probably transporting them to Australia instead,' said Jaz.

'Probably. Anyway, Burke and Hare decided it was easier to make their own dead bodies. So they killed all these people and sold them to a medical professor, who claimed afterwards he didn't know the bodies were murder victims. Yeah, *right*.'

'But the murderers were caught?'

'Yes, and Burke was hanged and they dissected his body in public and then turned his skin into leather and made it into souvenir wallets.'

'That's disgusting!'

'I know. Oh, I just remembered another "mort" word! *Mortsafe*. It was an iron cage that people would build around a grave to stop the body-snatchers getting to the coffin. Otherwise the family of the dead person would have to stand guard in the cemetery each night until the body rotted away.'

'I'm not sure I'd want my family to go to all that trouble,' said Jaz. 'I mean, once I'm dead, what does it matter what happens to my body? I'm not using it anymore. Better to have it educating medical students than rotting in the ground.'

'I suppose that's one way of looking at it,' said Rosy. 'But most people have a lot of *feelings* about death, don't they? What if families back then just didn't like the idea of their grandma's body getting mangled by medical students? Maybe she'd told them, "You make sure I stay in the ground where I'm buried, next to your grandpa!" and they all solemnly swore to respect her dying wish because they figured she'd haunt them for eternity if they didn't – Don't scoff! She *might* have! Anyway, it's her body. It's her decision what happens to it after she dies.'

'What if it's her decision not to donate any of her organs after she dies?' said Jaz. 'And meanwhile, sick people are spending their lives hooked up to oxygen tanks or kidney dialysis machines and little kids are dying waiting for a heart transplant?'

'I'm pretty sure they didn't do heart transplants in the 1800s, but yeah, I know what you mean. Dad has this friend who refuses to sign the organ donation card, because he reckons that if he signs it and then gets in an accident and they take him to hospital, the doctors won't bother trying to resuscitate him because they'll be desperate to take all his body parts. He *is* a bit paranoid, though. I think it's because he took a lot of drugs in the seventies, so they probably wouldn't want his body parts now, anyway. But there are also some people whose religion forbids them from donating any part of their body, even their blood. You can't force people to give up their religious beliefs.'

'Well, *I* think the needs of the living take priority over the dead,' said Jaz. 'I'm not saying that random people should be dragged off the street and forced to donate a kidney or a couple of litres of blood. But dead bodies aren't human beings anymore, so they ought to be used to give someone a new heart, or save someone's eyesight, or help with new research. What's more important – irrational superstitious beliefs or *science*?'

'If you choose science, that's *your* belief,' countered Rosy. '*I* might ask: What's more important, science or art? Like, I saw a documentary last year about people who'd agreed to have their bodies preserved with plastic after they died, to be put on display. *They* chose to donate their bodies to art, not science. Now, what was that exhibition called?' She'd turned back to Methuselah. 'Body Something ... Body Works? Body Worlds! Here it is. It's run by this German doctor, Gunther von Hagens.'

Jaz leaned in to examine his website. '*Is* that art? Or is it science? Look, he says his mission is to show how bodies work and how to stay healthy. So he sets up displays about how lungs get destroyed by smoking and what liver cancer looks like, that sort of thing.'

'But that isn't the main part of the exhibitions. People go to look at the whole bodies.' Rosy clicked on another page. 'See? There's a gymnast on a balance beam –'

'To demonstrate the muscles of the human body in action. Science.'

'And a woman kneeling, releasing some birds into the air, titled *Phoenix With Birds*. That's art. And a man ... holding up his peeled-off skin. Hang on, they're copying Vesalius! These muscle men are straight out of *De Humani Corporis Fabrica*!'

'Some of these poses are a lot weirder than Vesalius,' Jaz observed. 'They've got three skinless corpses sitting around a table, playing poker. And two of them are cheating.'

'Well, that's not very dignified,' said Rosy. 'Did the people who donated their bodies agree to be shown cheating at cards? I doubt it. They probably wanted to be javelin throwers or ballet dancers. It'd serve Gunther von Hagens right if their spirits came back to haunt him.'

'Rosy.' Jaz sighed. 'How many times? There. Are. No. Ghosts.'

Three sharp knocks rang out through the room, making both girls jump. Then the door slowly creaked open ...

'Hello,' said Alison. 'How's your project going?'

'Mum!' said Rosy, clutching her chest. 'You nearly gave me a heart attack! We thought you were a *ghost*.'

'No, I'm still alive, despite getting trapped in the longest departmental budget meeting in recorded history. Hello, you must be Jaz. I was just talking with your dad downstairs – no, no, don't worry, he said not to rush. He'll be at least another fifteen minutes packing up. Oh, is that von Hagens' exhibition?' Alison squinted at Methuselah's screen. 'I saw one of those in Amsterdam. Or was it Hamburg? Somewhere like that. I was at a medical conference just down the road, so a group of us went to have a look.'

'Was it art or science?' asked Rosy.

'Hmm ... Art, I think. I remember each of the bodies had a little card signed by von Hagens, explaining what the title of the display was and when he had "created" it – as though they were sculptures he'd built, not human beings he'd dissected.'

'So you didn't think it was educational at all?' said Jaz.

'Well, *I* didn't learn anything new from it,' said Alison. 'I suppose it might have been educational for some of the general public, but is there any evidence for that? It's not as though they made exhibition visitors do an anatomy quiz before and after the show, then a follow-up test six months later to see how much they'd remembered.'

'It says here that von Hagens calls his exhibition "edutainment",' said Rosy, turning back to the screen. 'He says he wants to entice people in with lots of fascinating exhibits, then make them think about death, because modern society tries to pretend death doesn't exist.'

'A worthy aim,' said Alison. 'But real death isn't plastic. It isn't clean and odourless, it's not anonymous and it's not arranged in artistic poses. This von Hagens is a showman, making money out of creating controversy – he had one of his preserved cadavers riding around on a bus when I was there. Well, good luck to him, as long as he gets informed consent from the body donors. But I don't think it's science.'

Her phone buzzed. 'Oh, I have to take this – it's one of my students,' said Alison. 'I'll be downstairs, Rosy. Good to meet you, Jaz.' She walked off, her phone clamped to her ear.

'I like your mum,' said Jaz quietly.

'Yeah, she's all right,' said Rosy. 'When she's not being a Mad Scientist, which is pretty much all the time. I wish she'd learn to cook, though, so we could have meals whenever we wanted in her flat. It's *hours* till they serve dinner in the refectory and I'm already starving – Hang on. Did you eat my apple?'

'*You* ate your apple, at lunch,' said Jaz, starting to gather up her papers. 'I ate *my* apple.'

'No, yesterday. Remember, I took an apple at lunch and then I said I'd eat it later? It was right here on my desk. But I had a huge dinner last night and wasn't hungry afterwards, and now it's gone.'

'The mummy must have eaten it,' said Jaz.

'Ha ha. Everyone knows mummies have their stomachs removed.' Rosy was on her knees, peering under the desk, then her bed. 'Okay, this is weird. It's vanished. I don't remember it being on my desk this morning, either.'

'Do ghosts have stomachs?' asked Jaz.

'It's easy for *you* to laugh about haunted rooms. *You* don't have to sleep in here tonight.'

Chapter Seven

'You don't have to sleep in here, either. You could spend the night in your mum's flat.'

'No,' said Rosy, getting to her feet and brushing off her knees. 'I'm not going to be chased out of my room. *And* I'm going to solve this mystery.'

'Use science,' suggested Jaz. 'Do an experiment. Try closing your window. Can I leave these library books here with you?'

'Huh?' said Rosy, still frowning around the room. 'Oh, yeah, sure.'

'I'll just take the books I need tonight,' said Jaz. 'That way, I can make a start on tomorrow's work. Can you print out the rest of the photos? Oh, and try to find out what you can about Dr Huxley. It might give us some clues about what the rest of his objects are. He must have been a student here – Rosy? Are you listening to me? What are you doing?'

Rosy was staring intently at the window.

'I'm thinking up an experiment,' she said.

CHAPTER EIGHT

'Science is nothing but trained and organised common sense.'
~ *T. H. Huxley*

It was three minutes to eight the next morning and Rosy was at her desk, eating a banana and scribbling away in her notebook. Glancing through the window, she saw Mr Singh's dusty ute roll up, right on time. However, instead of turning into the college car park, the vehicle continued down the road and disappeared.

'Odd,' remarked Rosy to the gargoyle. She returned to her notebook, wrote another sentence, frowned at it a while, then added a question mark. The ute reappeared, this time from the opposite direction. A minute later, Jaz herself turned up below Rosy's window, grinning broadly.

'Come down!' she called. 'I've got something to show you! You'll like it! It's *art*!'

Rosy tossed the banana peel in the bin, grabbed her notebook and ran downstairs.

'I saw it last month when Dad came here to deliver his landscaping quote and got lost,' said Jaz, tugging Rosy out of the college gates and down a side road. 'But I didn't realise the significance until last night.

You know how Vesalius showed that Galen was wrong about the human heart, how there weren't really any holes in it for blood to flow from one side to the other? Well, Vesalius still hadn't explained how blood did actually move around the body. That had to wait another eighty-five years for ... *this*.'

Jaz came to a halt on the footpath and, with a flourish, indicated a large brick building with an arched stone entranceway.

'Nice,' said Rosy, nodding. 'Art Deco. Probably 1930s. See that geometric metalwork in the windows and the –'

'No, the statues. That one there.'

'Oh, right. "Harvey". Hey, look, it's got one of those snake-on-a-stick medical symbols engraved into the plinth.'

'Well, that's because Harvey *was* a doctor, a really important one.' Jaz sat down on the low wall bordering the path and opened her own notebook. 'William Harvey, born in England in 1578, physician to King Charles the First, famous for writing *De Motu Cordis*, or "On the Motion of the Heart". He used science to demolish Galen's ideas about blood circulation.'

'Oh, good!' said Rosy. 'Go on.'

'Well, first – how much do you know about blood circulation? Do you know the difference between veins and arteries?'

'Yes. Veins are blue. Arteries are ... I don't know. Red? White? Deep beneath the skin so you can't see them? I know you're not supposed to cut them, otherwise blood gushes out and you bleed to death.

Chapter Eight

Oh – I guess that's why bloodletting always used *veins*, not arteries.'

'Right. Well, Galen thought that veins and arteries were parts of completely different blood systems. He thought the liver made blood that contained "natural spirits" and then veins carried this blood to all the organs and muscles of the body to nourish them. But he also thought there was another separate system, where the heart added air to blood to make "vital spirits". Then arteries pumped this "vital blood" to the different parts of the body, where it all got used up. None of the blood ever returned to the heart.'

'How did the heart add air to the blood? Hearts can't breathe in air.'

'Galen thought the pulmonary vein carried air from the lungs to the heart, as well as taking "sooty vapours" from the heart back to the lungs to get breathed out. But there were lots of problems with his theory. For one thing, the pulmonary vein is connected to the *left* side of the heart, but there are blood vessels taking blood away from the heart on the *right* side. How could blood get from the left to the right side of the heart when there's a thick wall down the middle? Vesalius couldn't find any holes in the wall. Neither could William Harvey. Harvey also couldn't see how the pulmonary vein could have spirit-filled air travelling in one direction and sooty vapours travelling in the opposite direction. When he cut the vein open, he found blood, not air. Plus, Galen didn't think the heart actively pumped blood around the body, but Harvey could see that it *did*.'

'I've got this wild, crazy notion,' said Rosy. 'I'm just throwing it out there, but is it possible that Galen was WRONG?'

'Anyone can say that a theory is wrong,' said Jaz. 'Harvey *proved* it was wrong. He calculated how much blood left the heart each time it pumped and how many times the heart pumped each hour. If Galen was right, and blood never returned to the heart after the body used it, then the liver had to make 540 pounds of blood each day. That's 245 kilograms, or about five times as much as I weigh. The average human body only holds about 5 kilograms of blood. If the liver really produced 245 kilograms of blood each day, all our blood vessels would explode from the pressure. Harvey realised that all the blood must be returning to the heart, then getting pumped around the body again, in a continuous circuit.'

'So Galen was vanquished by … maths.'

'What's wrong with maths?' said Jaz.

'Nothing,' said Rosy. 'Except for it being annoying and complicated and boring.'

'How can it be complicated *and* boring? Anyway, Harvey didn't just use maths and he didn't just do lots of observations of animals and humans. He did experiments. Want to see one? Hold out your arm.'

'Does this involve bloodletting?' said Rosy warily.

'All of your blood will stay in your body. It'll take about thirty seconds. There might be some temporary numbness, but no pain. I did it on my cousin last night and he showed no ill effects.'

Chapter Eight

'Your cousin Tej?'

'No, Rajindar. He was lifting weights in front of the TV and I could see his veins sticking out, so I asked if I could try it on him. He was still alive at breakfast this morning. But you really shouldn't do this experiment if you have any kind of disease affecting your blood circulation system. You don't, do you?'

'Not that I know of,' said Rosy. 'Okay, I hereby give informed consent for you to experiment on my arm.'

'Right,' said Jaz. 'Can I borrow your bandana? Now – I'm tying a tourniquet just above your elbow, tight enough to block all the arteries and veins. Notice that your upper arm is warm and starting to swell up, because blood is building up there. But your lower arm is getting colder and less pink.'

'Yep,' said Rosy, confirming this by feeling it with her free hand.

'Now I loosen the tourniquet a bit, just enough to let blood flow freely again in your arteries. They're deeper than the veins, you see. The veins are still blocked. Now blood is rushing into your lower arm, making it warm again. This shows that blood runs down your arm, from your heart, through the arteries. But notice how the veins in your lower arm are getting bigger? Squeeze your fist. See these little bumps along this big vein? Now, if I try to move blood up the vein with my finger, towards your heart, the blood moves easily. But the blood won't move *down* the vein, towards your hand.'

Jaz undid the tourniquet and handed it back to Rosy.

'Combined with all of Harvey's other information, this shows that arteries and veins are part of the same system, although they do different things. The heart pumps blood down to your hand through your arteries. Your hand uses up the oxygen and other things it needs from the blood. Then the blood, minus its oxygen, returns up the veins, back to your heart. Those little bumps in your veins are one-way valves, so blood in veins can only flow in one direction, back to the heart. The blood gets squeezed up the veins every time you move your muscles, like squeezing a tube of toothpaste.

'Oh, and the blood in the veins is purple because that's what colour blood turns once the oxygen's taken out of it. Then your heart pumps this purple blood to your lungs, which add oxygen to the blood and turn it bright red again. The blood goes back to your heart, and the heart pumps it back to your hand – and to all the other parts of your body, of course. Then repeat, over and over again.'

'Cool,' said Rosy, now tying the bandana around her other arm to see if the veins were the same size there. 'Well done, Harvey. Oh, wait, I have a question. How does the blood get from the end of the arteries in my hand to the start of the veins in my hand? Are the arteries and veins joined up, like two pipes stuck together? Because if they are, how does my hand get the oxygen out of the blood?'

'Good question. Harvey asked that, too. What happens is the arteries get thinner and branch out and

Chapter Eight

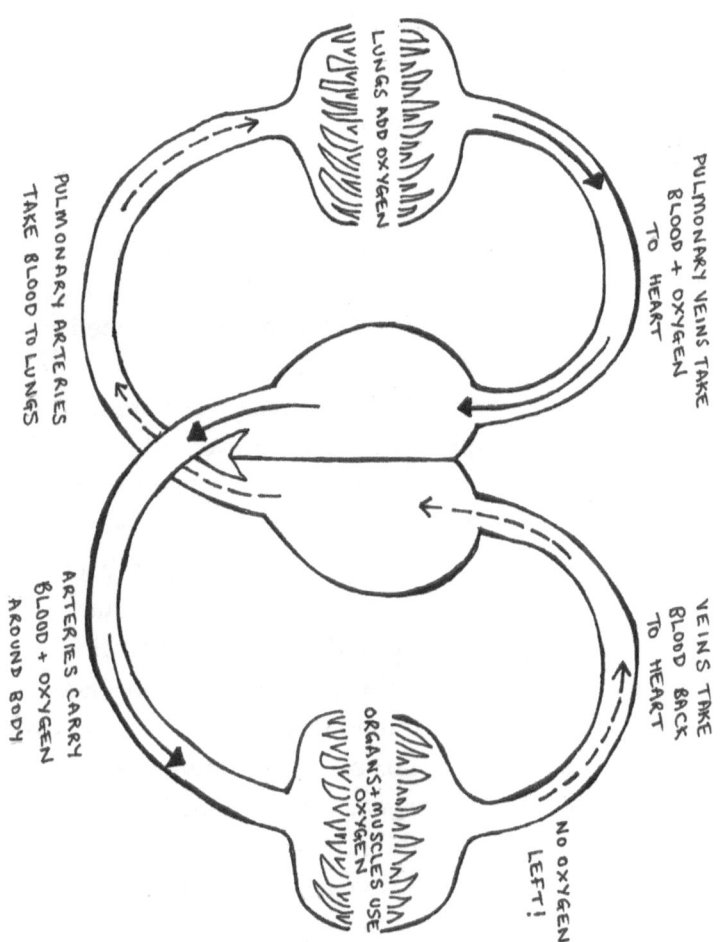

then there's a network of tiny capillaries that join up to the veins. Your hand can get oxygen out of blood in the capillaries, because capillary walls are incredibly thin. But here's how clever Harvey was. He couldn't actually see the capillaries because he didn't have a microscope, but he still worked out that they must exist. And that's why his statue is –'

'HEY! What do you think you're doing? Stop it!'

Rosy stopped poking her vein and looked up at Mohammad, who was marching towards them and gesticulating wildly at Rosy's tourniquet-wrapped arm.

'That's dangerous!' he cried. 'What are you, drug addicts or something? What would your parents say?'

Rosy and Jaz rolled their eyes at each other.

'Relax,' Rosy told him. 'We're not shooting up drugs. We're just doing a scientific experiment.'

'And *that*,' Jaz continued, turning her back on Mohammad, 'is why William Harvey's statue is outside the medical school. Because he revolutionised medicine by explaining the blood circulation system.'

'Hmph,' said Mohammad grumpily, watching Rosy untie her bandana. 'Harvey's only there because he was *English*. And *Christian*. What about Ibn al-Nafis, eh? *He* described how the lungs were connected to the heart, too – four hundred years before Harvey!'

'Yeah,' said Jaz, 'and Ibn al-Nafis also said that the main function of the heart was to heat the blood and thin it, and that blood was made in the liver, which are both wrong. Plus, he wasn't even translated into English till the twentieth century, so how could Harvey

Chapter Eight

have read his work? *Plus*, there were plenty of other people who figured out parts of the story. Harvey's own university lecturer, Fabricius, described one-way valves in veins, after Lusitano discovered them in 1547. Colombo and Servetus both wrote about how blood moved between the lungs and the heart. None of them proved it or put the whole story together. Who did? Oh, yeah – that was *William Harvey*.'

Mohammad retreated up the road, cowed into silence.

'You know, your brain is kind of scary,' Rosy told Jaz. 'Amazing, but scary.'

'Actually, there were lots of important Arabic medical discoveries,' Jaz confessed. 'I read up on it last night, after what Mohammad said yesterday. And not just Arabic, either – there were people from all different cultures and religions doing medical research. Lusitano was Jewish. It just happened to be Harvey who pulled all the facts about blood circulation together and made sense of it all.'

Jaz gave Harvey one last, respectful look, then turned to the statue on the opposite side of the entranceway. '"PASTEUR",' she said, reading the brass letters beneath the stern likeness of a gentleman with a lot of facial hair. 'I know he's a famous scientist, but I can't remember what exactly he did.'

'Invented pasteurised milk?' suggested Rosy. 'But don't ask me how that's different to normal milk. We should look it up, though – it's probably something important and medical.'

Jaz made a note in her book, then they started back up the road towards the college.

'Oh,' Jaz said suddenly, 'I forgot to ask about your room! Did it get haunted again? Did you do an experiment?'

'*Well*,' said Rosy, heaving a sigh. 'It turns out it's a bit more complicated than I thought, doing a scientific experiment. I mean, first you have to work out what your research question is. Then you have to do observations and background reading to figure out your hypothesis. And *then* you have to make sure you can test your hypothesis properly and predict what will happen if it's right ... I asked Mum for some advice, you see. It was a bit tricky – if I'd mentioned my room was being invaded at night, she'd have freaked out and made me sleep in her flat. Also, I try never to ask her anything about science, because I know I'll only understand about one word in twenty of what she says. But I took notes this time, see?'

Rosy flipped open her notebook and showed Jaz the first page. It said:

How to Use the Scientific Method To Answer a Question

Step 1: Write down the question you want to answer.
Step 2: Learn as much as you can about the subject. This is called Background information and observations.

Chapter Eight

STEP 3: Write your hypothesis. This should be a logical explanation that answers your question. MUST BE ABLE TO TEST HYPOTHESIS!

STEP 4: Do an experiment to test the hypothesis. Make sure you <u>control</u> for all <u>variables</u>. (WHAT?)

STEP 5: Analyse and interpret your results. (THIS HAD BETTER NOT INVOLVE MATHS!)

STEP 6: Does this prove your hypothesis is true? If it does, go to STEP 7. If hypothesis is not true, go back to STEP 3 and work out a better hypothesis.

STEP 7: Write up your results and publish them, so other scientists can repeat your experiment and show that your hypothesis is really, really true.

STEP 8: Become famous, win Nobel Prize, etc.

Then Rosy turned to the next page, where she'd written:

STEP 1: Who messed up the papers on my desk and stole my apple?!?

'That's two questions,' Jaz pointed out. 'You don't know for sure that whoever messed up your papers also stole your apple. They could be two completely unrelated events that just happened to occur on the same night.'

'Well, how likely is *that*?'

'Not very likely. But you can't assume anything in science.'

'I can assume some things,' said Rosy. 'Like, I'm assuming gravity works in my room because if I drop things, they always fall on the floor. So my apple probably didn't float out the window of its own accord.'

'Okay, you can assume things that other scientists have proven beyond reasonable doubt,' Jaz said. 'But you're still assuming a "who" was responsible. It could have been a "what" – like a breeze that suddenly blew up. Anyway, what happened last night?'

'I'm getting to that.' Rosy stopped in the middle of the road to cross out her question and write below it:

STEP 1
a) How did the papers on my desk get messed up on the night of the 8th of January?
b) Where did the apple on my desk go on the night of the 8th of January?

'I'm making it just that night, because I don't think my desk was touched last night,' Rosy explained. 'I took photos of my room before I went to bed and then as soon as I woke up, but I haven't had time to examine them carefully.'

'Did you leave your window open?'

'Yes, because it was boiling last night. *Again*. But anyway, that wasn't an experiment. I'm just gathering background information so I can work out a new hypothesis, because I decided my original hypothesis wasn't very good.'

She showed Jaz the next page, which said:

STEP 2
BACKGROUND INFORMATION AND OBSERVATIONS
MUMMIES
– Stomachs removed during mummification process, so a mummy wouldn't be able to eat my apple.
– Horus the Boy Mummy probably can't climb out of his locked glass case in museum. (Unless he has accomplice. NAOMI?!?) Also, probably can't walk very far, due to bandages wrapped tightly around legs, or climb through my tiny window, or unlock my door.

GHOSTS
– Can float through walls, so irrelevant if window open or not, or door locked.
– Do not eat apples.
– Probably can't move things by themselves.

'I don't think this has got anything to do with Naomi,' said Jaz. They'd reached the college by then and were climbing the narrow side staircase that led to Rosy's room. 'If it's a person, it's more likely to be Ms Boydell.'

'Hmm,' said Rosy, adding 'Boydell' to her notes. 'Anyway, I didn't have time to do more research, because I was really, really busy last night. I printed out all the photos of Dr Huxley's objects, which took ages, and I typed up your notes. Then we had dinner and Mum explained about the scientific method and I had to write all that down. And *then* I looked at all the photos in the foyer to see if Dr Huxley was in any of them, and of course, he was in the very, very last one.'

'Which photo?'

'A really old one of the swimming team, but the date was smudged. I'll show you when we go downstairs. He's listed as "Huxley, T., Med II".'

'So he *was* a doctor of medicine, not some other sort of doctor.'

'Yep. Anyway, then I typed "T. Huxley" into Methuselah and found heaps of websites about him.'

'Really? So he was famous! What did he do?'

Rosy unlocked her door, went over to the desk and picked up a printout.

'T. H. Huxley was a surgeon, biologist and professor, and received a number of prestigious awards for his scientific work,' she read. 'He was known for his passionate defence of Charles Darwin's theory of evolution and was a strong advocate for science education in schools and universities … Blah blah blah … Born in England, but visited Australia as a young man to do scientific research, and married a woman he met in Sydney. They had eight children. Oh, and he died in 1895.'

'Give me that,' said Jaz, snatching the paper away. 'This is about *Thomas* Huxley! Our doctor was *Timothy* Huxley.'

Chapter Eight

'Oh, yeah ...' said Rosy. 'I did wonder why the lawyers had taken so long to figure out his will and send his bequest here. Well, maybe the two Huxleys are related.' She sat down at her desk and turned on Methuselah. 'Meanwhile, let's find out all about pasteurised milk!'

'Not *now*,' said Jaz. 'We have to work out what the next object is. It's that big round flask in the wooden box.' She leaned over and started tapping at Methuselah's keyboard, which led to a minor scuffle, because Rosy was convinced that *she* was the only one able to handle Methuselah with the appropriate delicacy and tact.

'So, what do you think that liquid is?' Rosy said, once they were looking at the relevant photo. 'Some kind of medicine?'

'Maybe. Did it slosh around like water or was it thick like honey?'

Rosy thought for a moment. 'I don't remember it moving at all, but that's because we were carrying it so carefully. Maybe it's not a liquid at all. Maybe it's solid. Like ... wax or something? And is that a shadow on the front of the flask or some kind of label?'

'I think we'd better go and have a look at the real thing,' said Jaz.

'You can ask for the key at the office,' said Rosy, 'and I'll see if that Ms Boydell acts suspiciously.'

But Lynette was the only one in the office. She said the common room door was open and that they could keep the cabinet key for as long as they needed it. Up in the common room, Jaz unlocked the cabinet.

'I was right,' said Rosy. 'Look, there *was* a label on this flask, but most of it's worn off. See the round patch of glue ... Wait, there's a tiny bit of writing! Does this say "13"?'

'I think it's a capital "B".'

Rosy examined the writing more closely. 'That's handwritten in ink. This flask must be really old.'

'We'd better not try to take it out of the box, in case the glass shatters,' said Jaz. 'I'll just tilt the box slightly ... Well?'

'Yeah, it's some kind of thin liquid.'

'Medicinal tea?' suggested Jaz, as they both settled cross-legged on the rug to stare at the flask.

'Could be. Or what if that "B" stands for "blood"? Does blood turn that sort of clear orange-brown if you seal it up for hundreds of years?'

Jaz shook her head. 'I think it separates into layers. Anyway, there must be almost a litre of that liquid in there. If it was a blood sample, it'd just be in a little tube, wouldn't it?'

'It could be honey. That goes all runny in hot weather and it's the right colour. And honey has something to do with germs. Marcus is writing his thesis on honey.'

'He is *not*.'

'He is too. Mum told me when she introduced him. She said, "Marcus is doing important microbiological research into honey."'

'Oh. Well, then,' said Jaz, yielding at once. Clearly, she regarded Rosy's mum as an unquestionable source of wisdom.

Chapter Eight

They stared at the flask a bit more, but no other ideas transpired.

'We could go and ask Marcus,' said Rosy at last. 'Maybe germy honey was the cause of some horrible historical epidemic.'

'We can't bother him when he's working,' said Jaz.

'No, but we could just … go for a walk around campus and if we see him getting a coffee or something, we can ask him then.' The truth was, Rosy was feeling restless. She'd done a lot of heavy brain-work the previous night and now felt an irresistible urge to get back out into the sunshine. It *was* the summer holidays, after all. 'I mean, it's not as though we have any real clues for this thing,' she pointed out. 'It's still just a flask with some mysterious liquid in it. We're *stuck*. And my dad always says that whenever he feels stuck, he goes for a walk and then he gets inspired again.'

Jaz sighed and shifted her gaze to the next object, also encased in a velvet-lined box. 'What about this one, then?' she said. The tin sphere had several openings – one with a latched lid, one linked by a short pipe to a wider opening, and one attached to what appeared to be a crumpled brown paper bag. There was also a control knob on the side, its pointer able to swivel to different numbers etched into the metal. 'Some sort of medical instrument …' Jaz ventured, before trailing off in defeat. 'Okay, fine,' she said. 'A walk. Just for half an hour, though.'

After gathering up water bottles and hats and sunglasses, they set off up the road.

'Let's go this way,' said Rosy, pointing past the Sports Centre. 'I haven't been down this road before. Ooh, who's *that*?'

A gigantic bronze man stood by the side of the path, gazing resolutely into the distance. He sported a braided beard and a lot of interesting jewellery, and was clasping an unhappy-looking lion to his side with one of his massive, muscle-bound arms. Jaz brushed some leaves off his pedestal and read from the plaque.

'Gilgamesh, Assyrian King of Uruk during the Third Millennium BC. He went on a quest to seek immortality.'

'They were always trying to become immortal in the olden days, weren't they?' said Rosy. 'And it never worked out for them. You can't conquer Death. *I* could have told you that, Gilgamesh. That *lion* could have told you that, if you weren't squeezing all the breath out of the poor thing.'

Jaz frowned. '*You* were the one going on about the Elixir of Life yesterday.'

'I only said it was *possible*. But did the alchemists find any evidence for their hypothesis? Were their experimental results thoroughly analysed and interpreted? No, no and no. Really, Jaz, you need to start thinking logically and scientifically, like me.' Rosy dodged the leaf Jaz flicked at her and skipped off up the road. 'Anyway, who wants to live forever?' she continued, when Jaz caught up with her. 'I reckon it'd get dead boring after a couple of thousand years.'

'I don't want to live *forever*,' said Jaz. 'Just ... you know. Fifty or sixty more years. The normal amount.'

Chapter Eight

Then she fell silent and stayed that way, despite Rosy pointing out a number of interesting and amusing sights. It wasn't until they'd wandered past a cricket pitch, some sprawling red-brick buildings, a paved courtyard and a little white cottage, all of which were utterly deserted, that Jaz spoke again.

'Where to now?' she said. 'How about the library? I'd like to look inside, even if we're not allowed to borrow anything –'

But Rosy had drifted down a side lane, her attention snagged by the sign pointing to a shadowed doorway. 'I didn't know there was another museum here,' she said. 'The Macleay Museum … Now, why does that name sound so familiar?'

'It's a natural history collection,' said Jaz, reading the sign. 'Insects and fossils and things. Nothing to do with medicine. Come on.'

'No, wait,' said Rosy. 'I remember now! Macleay was a friend of Huxley's! Huxley wrote to him asking if there was a professor's job going here at this university!'

'That was *Thomas* Huxley,' said Jaz. 'The one who died in 1895. Come on, they'll have air conditioning in the library –'

But Rosy stood firm. 'I've got a feeling about this,' she said. 'We should take a look.'

'A *feeling*.' Jaz snorted. 'What happened to all your logical, scientific thinking?'

But Rosy had already pushed open the door and marched inside, so Jaz had no choice but to follow, grumbling under her breath as they were directed by a series of arrows up a lofty wooden staircase. Up and up and *up* they climbed, until they emerged into the dim space beneath the roof of the building.

'Cool,' breathed Rosy.

It was like stepping into the attic of some mad Victorian collector. The bleached skeleton of a whale dangled from the bare rafters, facing off the remains of a dugong, while the walls were lined with old wooden cabinets, each one crammed with curiosities. There were coiled-up snakes disintegrating in bottles of formaldehyde; rows of jewel-like beetles and butterflies skewered on silver pins; stuffed seabirds with beady glass eyes and bald patches where clumps of their feathers had fallen out; whorled shells and carved wooden masks and mats woven from palm leaves. There were old microscopes and astronomical sextants and cameras. There were also a lot of fuzzy brown photographs, mostly featuring men with serious beards.

'*All* museums should be like this,' declared Rosy, gazing at a moth-eaten ring-tailed possum. 'Lots of fascinating historical things, all jumbled together.'

'Pity none of them have anything to do with medicine,' said Jaz.

Rosy pointed at an enormous jar of pickled rats. 'What about them? They were probably killed during the bubonic plague epidemic!'

Jaz only shook her head and wandered off.

'Hey, Jaz,' whispered Rosy, some time later. 'Jaz! I've found a giant tapeworm in a bottle!'

Chapter Eight

When Jaz failed to reply, Rosy glanced round. Jaz was standing in the corner, staring into a storage area that had been roped off. 'Jaz?'

She went over to see what Jaz was gaping at – and her own jaw dropped.

'I don't believe it,' Rosy said. 'It *can't* be –'

'It is,' said Jaz hoarsely. 'It's exactly the same!'

'Didn't I *tell* you I had a feeling about –'

'Can I help you girls?' said a voice behind them, and they whirled around to find a tall, grey-haired woman giving them a quizzical look.

Jaz thrust a finger towards the object sitting on the benchtop. 'Where did you get *that*?' she demanded.

CHAPTER NINE

'Chance favours only the prepared mind.'
~ Louis Pasteur

Rosy hastened to apologise to the museum guide. 'Sorry, my friend's just a bit overexcited,' she said. 'It's only because we've got one exactly the same as that and –' Rosy suddenly clenched Jaz's arm. 'Jaz! It's still got its *label*!'

'Calm *down*,' whispered Jaz, shaking herself free and standing up straighter. 'Excuse me,' she said, turning to address the woman, who, fortunately, was looking amused rather than offended. 'Could you please tell us what's in that glass flask?'

'Flask?' said the woman, peering into the storage area. 'Oh, the one locked in the Perspex box? That's not actually part of our museum's collection. The Agriculture Honours students are organising an exhibition on Australia's rabbit infestation and they've borrowed a few things from the Pathology Museum. Just a moment –'

She unhooked the rope and went over to the bench. 'Shall I read out the label on this flask?' she asked.

'Yes!' cried Rosy and Jaz. 'Please,' added Jaz.

'The ink's faded, but it seems to say: "Bouillon. M. Pasteur. March 1888."'

'Pasteur?' said Jaz faintly.

'*Bouillon*?' said Rosy. 'That's French for broth. It's a flask of *soup*? Is it ... rabbit soup?'

The woman laughed. 'I've no idea. My area of expertise is flying foxes, not rabbits. Hang on, there's a file here.' She returned to the girls' side of the barrier, carrying some photocopied papers. 'Now you've got *me* curious. Let's see what these say.'

They gathered round to examine the papers.

'Here's a letter from the Director General of Public Health,' said the woman. 'It says, "In 1883, the rabbits had increased in such alarming proportions that the government of New South Wales offered a reward of £25,000 to anyone who could discover or provide a reliable method of destroying rabbits ... Offers came in freely from all parts of the world, amongst which was the scheme of Pasteur to kill them off by means of virulent cultures of Chicken Cholera." I assume they're referring to the famous Louis Pasteur there ... Ah, yes, here's a mention of the Pasteur Institute in Paris. It seems Louis Pasteur sent his nephew to Sydney with samples of cholera, as well as a dozen flasks of pure beef broth to use in their experiments. They grew their bacteria in broth in those days, of course.'

She looked over at the flask.

'Astonishing, isn't it?' she said. 'That broth is still as clear and unspoiled as when Pasteur sealed it inside that flask, one hundred and twenty-five years

Chapter Nine

ago. Well, it just shows how effective the process of pasteurisation is, doesn't it?'

Rosy sent Jaz a 'told-you-we-should-have-researched-that-this-morning' look (she was becoming quite fluent in Eyebrow Language), but Jaz didn't respond, clearly dumbfounded by all these amazing coincidences. Although, Rosy thought now, were they *really* so amazing? After all, the more you discovered about the world, the more you realised how connected everything was. And the more you learned, the more questions popped into your head, and the more likely it was that you went about, alert for any hint of an answer …

'And you said you own one of these flasks?' said the woman, now tapping the papers back into a neat pile.

'It's not really ours,' said Rosy. 'It was bequeathed to New College and our parents work there.' She elbowed Jaz, who pulled out the photo of the flask from her notebook and held it out to the guide.

'A pity the label's worn off,' the woman said, examining the image. 'That will make it difficult to authenticate. Your flask does look identical to this one, though. And even if it turned out Pasteur himself hadn't prepared yours, it would still be a fascinating medical artefact. Brings to mind his famous experiments on spontaneous generation, doesn't it? What a genius that man was! It's a shame his chicken cholera scheme didn't actually solve the rabbit problem, but then, even geniuses have their failures. Actually, they probably have even *more* failures than the rest of us, because they have to try out so many more new ideas …'

Back at New College, Rosy fired up Methuselah and Jaz started searching through her library books, most of which were now on the floor.

'You messed up my books,' Jaz complained. 'I had them all organised yesterday and now look at them ... Oh, here he is. Louis Pasteur, the Father of Germ Theory. I can't believe no one else had come up with that theory till the 1800s!'

'Well, germs are tiny, aren't they?' Rosy said. 'It's not as though anyone could see them crawling about on sick people – not until the microscope was invented, anyway. Although it says here that Varro wrote about invisible "animalcules" that caused diseases and that was back in 50 BC. He *meant* germs, even if he didn't call them that. Also, there was Fracastoro in 1546, Kircher in 1646, Andry in 1701 ... They all believed in germs.'

'None of them proved it, though, did they? And could you please stop saying *germs*? No one would ever guess you were the daughter of a microbiologist.'

'Ooh, sorry,' said Rosy. 'I *meant* to say teeny-weeny, incy-wincy, microscopic MICROBES. Hey, you know what Anton van Leeuwenhoek called them when he discovered them with *his* microscope? "Wretched beasties"!'

'Can we *please* get back to Pasteur? Now, listen. In the 1860s, he showed how microbes could spoil food. Oh, wait, I should be taking notes –'

Chapter Nine

'You talk, I'll type,' said Rosy, opening up a new document. 'I'll only have to type up your notes tomorrow, anyway.'

'– and that was how he came up with the idea of pasteurisation, which led to his famous discoveries about cholera and anthrax,' Jaz concluded, some time later. She glanced over. 'Have you got all that down?'

'Sure have!' said Rosy, a little too enthusiastically for Jaz.

'Let me see that,' she said suspiciously, tugging Methuselah towards her, then staring at his screen. 'Rosy! This is not what I said!'

'I may have done a bit of creative reinterpretation,' Rosy conceded.

Her document now read:

PROFESSOR PASTEUR'S AMAZING DISCOVERY
A Screenplay by Rosy Radford Smith
Featuring Historical Research by Jaz Singh

INT. SCENE – PROFESSOR PASTEUR'S LABORATORY, PARIS

PROFESSOR PASTEUR and his assistant, MONSIEUR BEAKER, are standing beside a bench covered with laboratory equipment. PROFESSOR PASTEUR opens his satchel and pulls out a thermos.

PROFESSOR PASTEUR

Mon Dieu! Madame Pasteur keeps giving me beef bouillon for lunch. I hate beef bouillon! But I can't tell her because I don't want to hurt her feelings.

MONSIEUR BEAKER

Please don't pour it down the sink again, Professor. The drain's blocked.

PROFESSOR PASTEUR

Hmm … I know! I will pour it into this glass flask, like so, and it will simmer away on top of this Bunsen burner, looking like one of my experiments. Then, if my dear wife comes in, she will suspect nothing –

MONSIEUR BEAKER

Professor, now you are making the whole lab smell like beef bouillon.

PROFESSOR PASTEUR

All right, I will seal the flask with a cork. *Voilà!* Now, go and fetch me a ham and cheese croissant from the café. Also, a nice glass of wine. If you see Madame Pasteur, pretend you're buying your own lunch …

SCENE DISSOLVE.
TITLE CARD: FIVE WEEKS LATER

PROFESSOR PASTEUR is standing at the benchtop when MONSIEUR BEAKER rushes into the lab.

MONSIEUR BEAKER

Professor, terrible news! The café has been closed down this morning by the food inspectors because the wine is sour, the butter is rancid and the cheese has gone off. There is no ham and cheese croissant for your lunch today, nor any wine!

Chapter Nine

PROFESSOR PASTEUR

Mon Dieu! Just when I finally talked Madame Pasteur into letting me buy my lunch at the café each day. And I'm hungry enough to eat a horse! Or even some beef bouillon. Hmm, that sealed flask of bouillon is still sitting here on the bench ...

MONSIEUR BEAKER

You can't eat that, Professor! It's been sitting there for weeks!

PROFESSOR PASTEUR

Do you want to listen to my tummy grumbling all afternoon? Let me just open the flask and see ... *Mon Dieu!* This bouillon is as fresh as when I sealed it five weeks ago! Taste this, Monsieur Beaker!

MONSIEUR BEAKER

[backs away]

Non, merci.

PROFESSOR PASTEUR

This is *très* interesting, Monsieur Beaker. You know how my arch-enemy, Félix Pouchet, thinks tiny animals just appear spontaneously in food if you leave it long enough? This flask demonstrates what a nincompoop he is! It is obvious that the tiny animals that spoil food are in the *air*. Heating this bouillon killed any tiny animals that had already fallen in it – then sealing the flask stopped new animals from falling in. That's why the bouillon hasn't gone bad.

But wait – I have a brilliant idea for a set of experiments! I will prove that the same microbes in spoiled food can also be found in the air! I will demonstrate that it's not the *air* that spoils food but the *microbes* in the air – yes, I will design a special flask with a swan neck that allows air in but traps microbes, and I will show that liquid kept inside that flask does not spoil! Also, I will explain to the café how to preserve their wine, beer and milk. If they boil it, it will ruin the flavour, but if they simply heat it to fifty-five degrees Celsius for a short time, as I did with my bouillon, it will kill the microbes and prevent spoilage!

MONSIEUR BEAKER

You are truly a genius, Professor. They will probably name this food preservation process after you. Forever after, it will be known as 'professorisation'.

PROFESSOR PASTEUR

But wait, I haven't finished! I think microbes do more than simply spoil food. I think they cause diseases and that each particular microbe causes its own specific disease. I have another brilliant idea. Quick, bring me three dozen chickens …

MONTAGE – Flasks bubble on Bunsen burners. Liquid is drawn up into syringes. MONSIEUR BEAKER chases chickens around lab. PROFESSOR PASTEUR heads out the door, carrying a surfboard.

SCENE DISSOLVE.
TITLE CARD: TWO WEEKS LATER

PROFESSOR PASTEUR
[re-enters lab, looking sun-tanned]

Chapter Nine

Okay, I am now back from my holiday, ready to resume my chicken cholera experiments. Bring me that cage of new chickens!

MONSIEUR BEAKER

Er ... There are only two new chickens left, Professor. You've used all the others. The chickens in that cage over there are the ones you injected with cholera last month.

PROFESSOR PASTEUR

Aren't they dead? They're supposed to be dead by now.

MONSIEUR BEAKER

Their feathers drooped a bit and they stopped eating for a while, but then they recovered.

PROFESSOR PASTEUR

This is *très* interesting, Monsieur Beaker. I injected them with that cholera that had been sitting around on the bench for days. I'd meant to throw that flask of cholera away, but I was too busy to tidy up the lab. Hmm ... I think I will now inject extremely strong cholera into *all* the chickens, both the old chickens that have recovered from their mild sickness and the new chickens, and see what happens ...

SCENE DISSOLVE.
TITLE CARD: ONE WEEK LATER

MONSIEUR BEAKER

Professor, all the new chickens are dead of cholera, but the old chickens did not even get sick this time! How can this be? They should all have died!

PROFESSOR PASTEUR

Let me think ... Aha! That first batch of cholera must have been weakened because it sat around for days on the bench. When I injected that cholera into the chickens, they caught only a mild version of the disease, but that made them immune to cholera forever after. So, later, when I injected them with the extremely strong cholera, they didn't get sick! Monsieur Beaker, do you know what this means? I have invented the first vaccine!

MONSIEUR BEAKER

Actually, Professor, for many years now, we have been using vaccines made from cowpox to protect people from smallpox. It's because cowpox is related to smallpox, but is a much milder disease, and so –

PROFESSOR PASTEUR

Yes, yes, I know all that! But most severe diseases don't happen to have a weaker cousin – the way smallpox is related to cowpox! I have invented the first safe vaccine that is made from the exact same germ that causes the disease. This has revolutionised medicine! From now on, all we have to do is identify the germ that causes a disease and then find a way to make the germ weaker – you know, by heating it, treating it with chemicals, leaving it sitting on a bench for a while to expose it to oxygen, something like that. Then we turn that weak germ into a vaccine and *voilà*! We prevent terrible diseases forever!

MONSIEUR BEAKER

You are truly a genius, Professor!

Chapter Nine

PROFESSOR PASTEUR

I know. Having vanquished chicken cholera, I will now develop a vaccine for the dreaded disease of anthrax. Bring me two dozen sheep, a goat and six cows …

'For a start,' said Jaz, 'the name of Pasteur's assistant was not *Beaker*. It was Charles Chamberland. And, more importantly –'

'More importantly, Pasteur showed that being tidy stops you making exciting discoveries,' said Rosy. 'If he'd thrown away the old cholera that was sitting on his bench, he'd never have come up with the idea of weakened-germ vaccines. And that's why I like to keep my room as messy as possible. You never know what you might discover in here. Anyway, go on, what did Pasteur do after he invented the anthrax vaccine?'

Jaz crossed her arms. 'I'm not saying anything else until you start typing normal notes.'

'Fine. Be boring. Okay, *okay*, I'm doing it …'

'Good,' said Jaz. 'Pasteur went on to make his greatest medical discovery, which was inspired by a terrible incident in his childhood. He'd witnessed a fatal attack on the village blacksmith by a mad wolf. Pasteur's father told him that the devil had got into the wolf, and that if God willed that you were to die, then there was nothing anyone could do about it … And no, Rosy, it was *not* a werewolf! The wolf had rabies, okay? Rabies makes animals go mad and bite people, then the people get infected, too, and they all die.

'But Pasteur decided he wanted to save people's lives, regardless of what God willed, and that's why he became a scientist. He was determined to find a way to stop rabies, so he found some rabid dogs, took samples of their saliva and tried to grow the rabies microbe in broth, except it didn't work. He couldn't even see any rabies microbes with his microscope. That's because, unlike cholera and anthrax, rabies is caused by a virus, rather than by bacteria.'

'What's the difference between viruses and bacteria?' asked Rosy.

'Um ... I'm not exactly sure,' said Jaz, turning to the index of her book.

'No, it's okay, I've found it,' said Rosy. 'They're both microscopic and cause diseases, but viruses are much tinier than bacteria and can only grow inside living animals. Thanks, Methuselah.' She patted his case. 'Go on, Jaz.'

'Well, Pasteur's assistant on this project – whose name, by the way, was Pierre Paul Émile Roux, not Beaker – worked out a way to grow the rabies virus by injecting it inside dogs' brains.'

'*Living* dogs? Oh, the poor things!'

'I know, but Pasteur didn't have any other method. It was the only way to stop rabies, which was a really, really awful disease, for people and animals. It caused convulsions and frothing at the mouth and paralysis and insanity and the victims always died in agony. Anyway, Pasteur finally managed to weaken the virus and turn it into a vaccine and it worked perfectly on

Chapter Nine

the laboratory dogs. Only he couldn't test the vaccine on healthy people, because if it didn't work, the people they'd tested it on would die horribly. Then, one day in 1885, a woman burst into the lab. A rabid dog had viciously attacked her nine-year-old son, Joseph Meister. Poor little Joseph was covered in bites and blood and foam. He was going to die in the most terrible way. She begged Pasteur to help her child. Pasteur warned her that his vaccine had never been tested on humans, but she was willing to try anything. And so for the next ten days, he gave Joseph a series of injections.'

Jaz closed her book.

'And?' said Rosy, leaning forward when Jaz didn't say anything else. 'Come on, what happened then?'

'Oh, I thought maybe it was boring you ... Ow! Yes, of course, it worked! Joseph's life was saved and Pasteur went on to vaccinate thousands of people against rabies, including some Russian villagers who'd been bitten by a mad wolf. The Russian Tsar was so grateful that he gave Pasteur a hundred thousand francs to establish the Pasteur Institute for medical research and Joseph Meister ended up working there after he grew up.'

'Aw, that's a nice story,' said Rosy. 'I liked that one. Well, it was terrible about the poor dogs being injected with rabies, but at least they didn't die in vain.'

'Mmm,' said Jaz, who'd reopened her book. 'Hey, have you ever heard of Robert Koch? This is really interesting ...'

And she remained glued to the book for some time, resisting all of Rosy's attempts to prise her fingers off it when they went downstairs for lunch.

'Did you know that it was Koch, not Pasteur, who was the first to identify the bacteria that caused anthrax?' said Jaz. 'Koch also discovered the bacteria that caused tuberculosis, which killed thousands of people each year by spreading from cows to people through infected milk –'

Rosy paused, her glass of chocolate milk halfway to her lips.

'But fortunately, pasteurising milk kills all the tuberculosis bacteria in it,' said Jaz. 'Also, Koch discovered the bacteria that caused cholera – human cholera, that is, not the chicken cholera that Pasteur worked on. But even then, in the 1880s, people refused to accept that bacteria could cause diseases. There were all these doctors and professors who still believed in the miasma theory.'

She waited for Rosy to ask what the miasma theory was, which Rosy obediently did.

'They thought diseases like cholera and the plague were caused by rotting things giving off a foul smell, then people breathing in this poisoned "miasma",' Jaz explained. 'It sort of made sense, because more people tended to get sick in the filthy areas of the cities, which smelled horrible. But there was this one doctor in London, John Snow, who was convinced that the miasma theory was wrong, and this was decades before Pasteur and Koch's work.

Chapter Nine

'Dr Snow studied the cholera epidemic of 1849 and pointed out that if it had really been spread by gas, then the entire population should have got sick. After all, everyone breathed in the same air, but only certain people came down with cholera. Besides, cholera didn't even affect the lungs – it attacked the intestines, which suggested it was caused by something that people swallowed. Then, when another epidemic started in 1854, Dr Snow did some very clever detective work …'

'Will you stop doing that?' said Rosy impatiently. 'Just tell me what happened!'

'I have to read what the clever detective work actually *was* … Oh, right. Well, he got a map of Soho, the district where he worked, and coloured in every household where someone had died of cholera. He noticed that right in the middle of those coloured-in houses was a water pump in Broad Street. Then he interviewed as many people in the neighbourhood as he could and found that most of the cholera victims had used that pump for their drinking water. There was a prison nearby where no one got sick – but they had their own well. And none of the workers at the Broad Street brewery got sick because they drank beer, not water. Dr Snow realised that the water from the pump had been contaminated with raw sewage –'

Rosy gagged. 'I am trying to eat lunch here, you know.'

'Sorry. Anyway, he persuaded the authorities to take the handle off the pump so that no one could use it and the cholera epidemic ended. Then he convinced

Parliament to improve the city's drains so the sewage would –'

'If you insist on talking about microbiology all through lunch, could it at least be a story that doesn't put me off my food?'

Jaz flipped through the pages. 'Okay, then, you'll like this one. You know how Pasteur used broth to grow bacteria? Well, the problem was that it's not very good for growing pure forms of bacteria. All sorts of other bacteria can end up growing inside the liquid and they get mixed up together, so you can't be sure exactly which bacteria you're using in your experiments. But one day, Koch happened to notice that someone had left a slice of boiled potato sitting on a bench in his lab. There were little blobs of colour growing on the potato and when he looked at each blob with his microscope, he saw that each colour was a different pure colony of bacteria.

'He realised that the best way to grow bacteria wasn't in liquid, but on a flat, solid surface, so the bacteria stayed in the one place and didn't get mixed up. Unfortunately, most bacteria didn't grow well on sliced potatoes. He tried adding gelatin to broth to make jelly, but that didn't work either, because something in the bacteria dissolved the gelatin, and anyway, jelly turns to liquid at the warm temperatures that bacteria like. Then a lab assistant, Fanny Hesse, said that when she wanted to set her jams and jellies at home, she used agar, which comes from seaweed. It turned out that agar mixed with broth was perfect for growing

Chapter Nine

bacteria, especially when it was set in a flat, shallow dish invented by Julius Petri, another assistant.'

'Hey, and microbiologists still use Petri dishes!' said Rosy. 'I remember when I was little, Mum brought some home so I could take swabs of my fingers and the TV remote control and the door handle and stuff. And then we put the Petri dishes near the heater and all these disgusting blobs of germs started sprouting up on the agar. I think it was meant to teach me to wash my hands more often. It worked, too.'

'Well, anyway, Koch was a genius. He should really be more famous than Pasteur. Koch developed all these techniques for adding dyes to bacteria on glass slides so you could see them properly with a microscope, and he was the first to photograph bacteria, and his team went on to discover the microbes responsible for diphtheria, typhoid, pneumonia, leprosy, bubonic plague and tetanus. But he's best known for thinking up Koch's Postulates –'

'Which were used to prove that a particular microbe was the cause of a particular disease,' said Rosy. 'Thereby destroying the miasma theory and changing microbiology forever.'

Jaz gaped across the table at her. 'How did you know that?'

'Elementary, my dear Watson,' said Rosy. 'I can read upside down.'

'*I'm* Sherlock Holmes, not you,' said Jaz, clutching the book to her chest to hide the pages. 'And I bet you can't list the four postulates!'

'As if Sherlock cares about postulates. Learning postulates off by heart is the sort of thing *Watson* would do. You're totally Watson. I bet you even want to be a doctor like him when you grow up –'

'Shh!' hissed Jaz, glancing about. 'Keep your voice down!'

'What? Why?' said Rosy. 'Are you looking for your dad? He's out in the foyer.'

'Oh,' said Jaz, relaxing. 'I thought he was still in the kitchen.'

'So you *do* want to be a doctor, then?' This wasn't exactly shocking news to Rosy, so she couldn't imagine it would come as any surprise to Mr Singh. Besides, he seemed quite proud of his daughter's braininess, from what Rosy had seen. 'What's wrong with that?'

'Nothing. I just don't want my dad to hear because … um, because I might not be smart enough to get into medical school.'

Rosy gave a disbelieving snort.

Jaz glared at her. 'I might not be! And even if I got in, it'd take years and years to qualify as a doctor and … Look, my dad doesn't like talking about stuff that far into the future, okay? Anything could happen before that.'

'*Anything could happen?*' said Rosy. 'Like what, we could all get squashed by a giant meteorite or eaten by aliens or –'

'Now you're being ridiculous. Come on, have you finished eating? Let's go upstairs and have another look at Dr Huxley's next object. I've got some ideas about what it might be.'

Chapter Nine

Actually, Rosy was sure Jaz didn't have a clue about the next object. She'd simply been trying to change the subject, but Rosy knew when to take a hint. And then they got so busy organising the research they'd already done and checking all their facts and printing everything out on nice paper that before they knew it, it was time for Jaz to go home and Rosy had almost forgotten that whole weird conversation.

Unfortunately, she'd also forgotten to retrieve her favourite pen from where she'd left it in the Senior Common Room, but Rosy's mum turned out to have her own key. It did mean that Rosy had to explain why she and Jaz had been in there in the first place – that they were researching Dr Huxley's collection in order to make labels for each object – although she avoided the bit where they'd managed to lose all of Dr Huxley's notes in the turtle pond and up a gum tree. She figured her mum would be too distracted by Pasteur's flask to ask any tricky questions, and she was right.

'Fascinating,' murmured Alison, gazing into the cabinet. 'I spent a few months at the Pasteur Institute when I was a post-grad student. There was some amazing work being done there. Did you know that's where they discovered the virus that causes AIDS?'

'Really?' This reminded Rosy of something she'd been pondering. 'Hey, Mum. Which are worse, bacteria or viruses? Like, which have killed more people?'

'What, throughout history? Well ... bacteria cause plague – and that's killed at least a hundred million people since the Middle Ages. In recent times, though, it's probably been viral infections that have been deadlier. About fifty million died in the 1918 influenza pandemic, you know, and then there were all those millions of people killed by smallpox, polio, hepatitis, measles ... and AIDS, of course, and now there's Ebola and Zika.

'The problem with viral diseases is that it's so difficult to find a cure for them. Antibiotics can kill bacteria, but viruses work by getting inside human cells and changing them. Any medicine that kills the virus is probably going to be so toxic, it'll kill the person's cells as well, and it's really hard to stop a virus replicating itself once it's infected someone. There are vaccines to prevent some viral diseases, but viruses mutate so quickly and can jump from one species to another. That's why there are so many different types of flu and why we need to make a new flu vaccine each year.'

'Okay, viruses are worse than bacteria,' decided Rosy. 'Do you reckon viruses are the main cause of death now? Oh, no, wait, that's probably cancer or something.'

'Well, viruses can cause cancer, too.'

'No way! You can't *catch* cancer.'

'Of course you can. Lots of viruses cause cancer. Hepatitis viruses can cause liver cancer. Epstein-Barr virus can cause lymphoma. Human papillomavirus causes several types of cancers, including cervical cancer in women. Why do you think you and all the other girls in your class were given the Gardasil vaccine last year? That vaccine was to protect you against the human papillomavirus. There's even a hypothesis

Chapter Nine

that some mental illnesses, like schizophrenia, can be caused by Borna virus.'

'Right, that's it! Viruses are the worst thing ever!'

'Oh, they're not all bad,' said Alison. 'Some viruses can infect bacteria, so we use them in the lab to study how bacteria work. There's a lot of exciting research now trying to use viruses as medicine, to kill bacteria when antibiotics don't work or to get inside cancer cells to destroy them.'

'Hmm,' said Rosy. 'All right, then. When I rule the world, maybe I'll allow *some* viruses to exist –'

'What's this thing?' interrupted Alison, peering at the object sitting beside the flask.

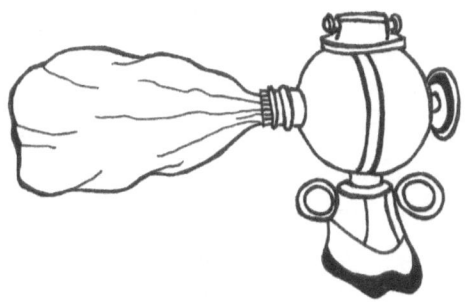

'Oh, that,' said Rosy. 'That's a weird tin contraption. I want to figure it out before Jaz does, though. Do you have any ideas?'

'Let's see,' said Alison, scanning the shelves. 'You've got the skeleton picture, then Pasteur's flask ... So, logically, this next artefact should have something to do with surgery.'

'*Surgery*? How do you figure that out?'

'Well, that was the next step in the history of medicine. First they had to understand how the human body is put together – that's anatomy. Then they had to figure out how to do operations without the patient dying of an infection afterwards – that needed microbiology. Did you know Pasteur was one of the first to tell surgeons to boil their instruments to stop infections spreading?'

'Okay, but that tin thing doesn't look like anything you'd use in an operation. It's not a scalpel or clamps or anything. It looks like … one of those old-fashioned metal diving helmets. For a very tiny diver with a head the size of a tennis ball, who wants to walk around on the bottom of a goldfish bowl.'

'There you go. Perhaps that wide opening is a mouthpiece. Because apart from stopping patients dying of infections, surgeons also had to figure out how to stop their patients going into shock from the agonising pain. Remember what happened when you had your tonsils removed?'

'No, because I was … ASLEEP! Is *that* what this is, some sort of device for breathing in sleepy gas?'

'Also known as general anaesthetic, and yes, possibly. What's that engraved into the metal?'

'It says "COLLIN", I think. The rest is too scratched to read. Wait, there's a number as well!'

'That should be enough to –' began Alison.

But Rosy was gone. Out the door, racing down the corridor, heading for Methuselah.

CHAPTER TEN

*'Science moves, but slowly, slowly,
Creeping on from point to point'*
  ~ Alfred, Lord Tennyson

'I don't believe it!' said Jaz the next morning. 'I mean, I *do* believe it, but ... it's just really weird, that's all.'

'You're telling me,' said Rosy, studying the papers scattered over her floor. The Midnight Visitor had struck again.

'And there *definitely* wasn't any breeze last night,' Jaz said. 'They were saying on the news that this is the longest heat wave the city's experienced in twenty-five years.'

'I know,' said Rosy. 'I thought about going down to Mum's flat because she has air conditioning, but I was too tired to get out of bed. And the next thing I knew, it was morning and I found all *this*.'

'So you didn't hear anything? No suspicious noises?'

'Nothing. And my door was locked.'

'Your apple's gone from the desk, too,' observed Jaz.

'No, I didn't have an apple on my desk last night, so I don't think the apple has anything to do with it. And now I'm really annoyed I didn't take a photo before I went to bed. Now there's a gap in my data! But I was just so sleepy, I forgot. I stayed up late, you see, doing research, plus Mum made me tidy up my room, although I couldn't be bothered to –'

Rosy broke off and stared at the bin, now lying on its side in a welter of crumpled tissues, pencil shavings and lolly wrappers.

'What?' said Jaz.

'I couldn't be bothered emptying the bin,' said Rosy slowly, 'because I'd have to take it all the way downstairs. Jaz – a new, improved hypothesis is forming in my brain!'

Jaz arched an eyebrow. 'And are you going to tell me what it is?'

'Not yet. I need to do some background research first.'

'Right. Well, can we tidy this up, then?'

'Yeah, I only left it like this to show you,' said Rosy. 'I've taken a photo of it.' They started to clean up the mess. 'Oh, and by the way,' Rosy added, 'I figured out what our next object is.'

'What?' cried Jaz. 'I don't believe it! I mean, I do, but – What is it?'

'Here,' said Rosy, and she picked up some papers from the floor and handed them to Jaz. They read:

A BRIEF HISTORY OF SURGERY
By Rosy Radford Smith

People have been using surgery to treat injuries and illnesses since the Stone Age. Prehistoric surgeons were especially fond of drilling holes in their patients' skulls with sharp stones and there's evidence that some of those poor people actually *survived* the procedure, although how, I don't know. Ancient civilisations, including the Sumerians, Egyptians, Indians and Romans, went on to develop metal surgical instruments and fancier techniques, but unfortunately, no one got around to inventing antibiotics or anaesthetics, so having surgery still wasn't very enjoyable or effective.

Ignoring the extreme pain, blood loss and lethal infections, surgeons continued to hack away at people throughout the Middle Ages. The most famous surgeons of this time, Cosmas and Damian, were twin brothers who became the patron saints of medicine after they successfully sawed off a living man's gangrenous leg and sewed in its place the leg of a dead man. (Note: According to this story, Cosmas and Damian also miraculously survived being crucified, stoned and shot with arrows during their martyrdom, dying only after their heads were cut off, so make up your own mind about how true it is.)

There were attempts to make surgery less painful by drugging patients with hemlock, opium, mandrake root and wine, but often the patient failed to wake up again afterwards. Praying and singing hymns during an operation were also popular but not very effective. Likewise 'mesmerism', which meant trying to hypnotise the patient into feeling no pain. Surgeons became known for their speed (for instance, in the 1830s, James Syme was able to amputate a leg in ninety seconds), but obviously, they couldn't do any really complicated surgery until general anaesthetics were invented.

The first of these was nitrous oxide. In 1795, Humphry Davy noticed that inhaling this gas caused dizziness and giggling, so he suggested it might be useful for relieving pain during operations. There followed a craze for 'laughing gas' at fun fairs and parties, but it wasn't till 1844 that Horace Wells, an American dentist, decided to try it as an anaesthetic while having his own tooth yanked out. He felt no pain at all! This could have led to something exciting, except the machine he built to administer the gas to dental patients malfunctioned during its first demonstration, everyone else lost interest, and Horace Wells went mad and died.

There was also a more powerful gas called ether, which was discovered by Valerius Cordus in 1540. Paracelsus tried it on chickens and reported that it made them 'undergo prolonged sleep' and 'awake unharmed', but for some reason (maybe because other doctors found him so annoying), no one paid any attention to this information for hundreds of years.

Chapter Ten

However, in the 1840s, William E. Clarke, Crawford Long, William Morton and John C. Warren successfully used ether in America for minor surgeries. Then a famous Scottish surgeon, Robert Liston, amputated a patient's leg with the help of ether. (It took him twenty-eight seconds. Not for nothing was he known as 'the fastest knife in the West End'. Incidentally, he once accidentally chopped off the fingers of his surgical assistant, who then died of gangrene.) Ether became a popular anaesthetic, but it did have a few problems. Firstly, it caused sore throats and coughing. Secondly, it made lots of patients vomit. Thirdly, it was highly flammable – and many doctors in those days operated by candlelight.

But then an alternative appeared! In 1847, a Scottish professor called James Young Simpson and some of his doctor friends were experimenting in his dining room, when they decided to try sniffing a liquid called chloroform. Some time later, they all woke up dazed and confused under the table, tangled up with the chairs. Dr Simpson then successfully used chloroform in surgery and to help women give birth, but he also had a lot of fierce arguments with religious leaders, who said that any kind of pain relief, especially during childbirth, was unnatural and immoral. However, Queen Victoria used chloroform when she gave birth to Prince Leopold in 1853 and described the experience as 'delightful', so it became very popular. (By the way, the doctor who administered the chloroform to her was John Snow, famous for his cholera detective work in Soho. He was a very busy man.)

Alas, chloroform was so powerful that it often killed patients! So, it was back to ether. Fortunately, in 1907, Louis Ombredanne invented a special device that made ether much easier and safer to use for surgery. The Ombredanne inhaler, which you can see in this cabinet, consists of a metal sphere with an opening at the top for inserting a sponge soaked in liquid ether. At the bottom is a wide mouthpiece for breathing in the ether fumes. The swivel gauge at the side allowed the doctor to control how much air or ether the patient was breathing in. The bag attached to the other side was a reservoir to hold the air-and-ether combination that the patient breathed out (and no, that's not a paper bag – it's a caecum bladder, made of animal intestines). The French instrument maker, Collin, made this particular inhaler in about 1910. The Ombredanne inhaler was used throughout Europe until the Second World War, and to this day, doctors use ether during surgery.

'That's really interesting,' said Jaz, putting down the papers. 'Because *I* was reading up on surgery last night, too.'

'Great minds think alike.'

Chapter Ten

'Well, I wasn't really thinking about this object. I was just wondering how long it took for hospitals to accept Pasteur and Koch's evidence and to start using antiseptic techniques to stop infections. Did you know that for a long time, surgeons actually *encouraged* pus to develop in wounds?' Jaz opened her notebook and began riffling through the pages. 'And guess who came up with the idea of pus being a good thing?'

'Not Galen again!'

'Yep. Where did I ... Oh, here it is. Borgognoni argued against this idea of "laudable pus" in 1267 in his book, *Chirurgia*, saying it was better to clean wounds, stitch them up and cover them with wine-soaked bandages. The alcohol in the wine would probably have helped disinfect the wound. But most doctors seemed to ignore this advice. Plus, they did all sorts of horrible things to stop bleeding, like sealing blood vessels with red-hot irons and pouring boiling oil on wounds.'

'Could you move on to the bit where they stopped being so disgusting?' said Rosy, wrinkling her nose.

'Okay, you'll like Ambroise Paré. He was a sixteenth-century French military surgeon who usually followed the awful advice in the medical textbooks of the time. But one day, he ran out of boiling oil to pour over the soldiers' gunshot wounds, so he decided to use an ointment made of egg white, oil of roses and turpentine. He was amazed to see that the men treated with boiling oil ended up with painful, inflamed wounds the next day, while the men who'd had the ointment felt much better. He wrote, "At this, I resolved never again cruelly to burn poor people who had suffered shot wounds" and his motto became, "I bandaged him and God healed him". Oh, and he also developed a method of tying off blood vessels to stop patients bleeding to death during limb amputations.'

'Good work, Ambroise!' Rosy pulled Methuselah closer and began typing notes.

'But infection was still a huge problem, even three hundred years later, especially in hospitals. Lots of surgeons worked in blood-soaked gowns and didn't even wash their hands before starting an operation. A hospital doctor in Vienna called Ignaz Semmelweis became convinced it was doctors themselves who spread disease. He noticed that mothers in a maternity ward staffed by medical students had a twenty-nine per cent death rate from puerperal fever – also called childbed fever – but mothers looked after by midwives in the next ward had only a three per cent death rate.

'He knew those medical students often went straight from doing autopsies on diseased corpses to delivering babies. Their professor had actually died of an infection after he accidentally cut his finger during an autopsy – and Semmelweis realised that the infection looked exactly the same as the one the new mothers were dying from. So in 1847, Semmelweis told all his staff to wash their hands in chlorinated water before delivering babies and the death rate for mothers fell to below one per cent.'

'And then he won lots of awards and became rich and famous?'

Chapter Ten

'No, because his doctor colleagues refused to believe that puerperal fever was contagious or that they were responsible for spreading the disease. Then Semmelweis went mad and died.'

'Okay, this is depressing.' Rosy slumped forward, her chin on one hand.

'No, it's not, because in spite of the stupid doctors, hospitals started to become more sanitary. Florence Nightingale and her nurses took over a military hospital during the Crimean War in the 1850s and reduced the death rate from forty per cent to two per cent, mostly by cleaning up the wards. Mind you, Florence Nightingale didn't believe in bacteria, either – she supported the miasma theory.

'There *were* some surgeons who paid attention to Pasteur, though, like Joseph Lister. In the 1860s, he worked out that carbolic acid killed the bacteria that caused gangrene. So he washed himself with carbolic solution before operations, sprayed carbolic acid vapour around the operating theatre and dressed his patients' wounds with bandages soaked in carbolic acid. And it worked. The number of his patients dying of infections after surgery dropped from forty-six per cent to fifteen per cent.'

'The other doctors couldn't argue with that, could they?' asked Rosy, straightening up again.

'Some of them did. They just couldn't accept that they were wrong. And the others complained that carbolic acid irritated their skin, but that was okay, because a Prussian surgeon called Ernst von Bergmann worked out better ways of keeping operating theatres clean and, also, how to sterilise instruments using steam. And then surgeons started using face masks and rubber gloves and gowns, so eventually they could do really complicated operations, like heart surgery, without the patient routinely dying of an infection afterwards.

'They did go a bit too far, though. Like, now that surgery was much easier and safer, doctors suddenly decided that kidneys that were too low caused back pain, so they invented an operation called "hitching up the kidneys". And if patients had any kind of stomach pain at all, they'd immediately have their appendix taken out. Rich people in the 1930s would even have their appendix removed before they left on a long cruise, just in case they got a sore stomach while they were away from their doctor –'

'Slow down,' said Rosy, who'd been typing as Jaz spoke. 'I'm still on rubber gloves and face masks. Okay ... Now, what was that about hitching up kidneys? How could doctors get away with that sort of ridiculous stuff?'

'Well, doctors were like God, weren't they? No one ever questioned them. They were the experts. Patients went along with whatever the doctor said.'

'Even if it didn't actually make the patients feel any better?'

'Maybe their back pain *did* improve after their kidneys were shifted,' said Jaz thoughtfully. 'I mean, sometimes back pain goes away by itself if you stay

Chapter Ten

in bed for a while. And then I suppose the doctors would say it must have been the kidney operation that had fixed the problem. And if the patient *didn't* feel any better, the doctors would just ... ignore that information? No, I don't get it. I mean, doctors were using science to work out how to kill bacteria, so why didn't they use it to figure out which operations were useful and which weren't?'

'Bacteria are much easier to study, though,' Rosy pointed out. 'You spray carbolic acid on them and then look at them under a microscope to see if they're dead or not. Simple. Humans are a lot more complicated.'

'I know,' said Jaz, with a sigh. 'So, are we finished with surgery now? What's Dr Huxley's next object?'

CHAPTER ELEVEN

'Science is much more than a body of knowledge. It is a way of thinking.'
~ Carl Sagan

'Next are the mysterious fragments of old print,' said Rosy. 'Here, I enlarged the photo, not that it helps much. I can read all the letters – I can even work out a few words at a time – but a lot of it's complete nonsense.'

'This sentence makes sense,' said Jaz, pointing at one section. '"Two others had each two oranges and one lemon given them every day." But then the next bit is: "Thefe they eat with gree-dinefs"!'

'I think it must be from an old book. See here at the top, "Chap. IV."? That could be Chapter Four.'

'And then the words next to that might be the title of the book,' said Jaz. 'There's a smudged bit, then "of the f curvy."'

'Could that be the author's name? You know, like Andreas Vesalius had his name at the top of each page in his anatomy book? "F. Curvy." Frederick Curvy? Francisco Curvy. Fiona Curvy …'

'There are too many "f"s on this page,' said Jaz, frowning at it. 'Wait, look at this – "hofpital-furgeon".

That has to be *hospital-surgeon*! They're writing an "f" every time they should put "s"!'

'No, they're not. See, there are plenty of examples of "s". "Oranges and lemons", "patients", "currants" ...'

'Oh, you're right,' said Jaz. 'Hey, this looks like a list of ingredients: "garlic, muftard-feed, *rad. raphan.* balfam of *Peru*, and gum myrrh".'

'Maybe it was a secret recipe for medicine and that's why they wrote it in code. Want to go down and have a look at the real thing? I've got Mum's key to the Senior Common Room.'

But the fragments of yellowed paper, mounted on stiff card and framed under glass, revealed no further information. Rosy and Jaz were still kneeling in front of the cabinet, tossing unhelpful suggestions at each other, when they were interrupted by an unfamiliar voice.

'Dear *me*, tutors at this college are getting younger and younger each year!'

Rosy and Jaz whipped around to find a white-haired lady, much smaller than the voice suggested, leaning on a walking stick in the doorway. 'Oh, don't be alarmed,' the old lady continued, hobbling into the room. 'I shan't inform the authorities about your blatant act of trespass – provided you do me a *tiny* favour. Look behind that sofa, will you, and tell me if you detect a pair of gold-rimmed spectacles. No? Then perhaps one of you would be so kind as to peek underneath that table over there ...'

After a prolonged search, Jaz located the missing spectacles on top of a bookcase.

Chapter Eleven

'Oh, yes, I was sure they must be in here,' said the old lady, putting them on and blinking around the room. 'We had a little cocktail party to celebrate my retirement at the end of last semester and things became rather boisterous. Quite a few objects were misplaced. But now I can see you properly – and also examine this very interesting display of yours. Ah! Now, *that* object reminds me of my recent trip to Cairo.'

'We haven't put the labels up yet,' Rosy said, 'but that's an Eye of Horus healing amulet.' And she and Jaz went on to explain the significance of various other objects in the cabinet.

'How intriguing!' said Dr Bennet. (They had all introduced themselves by then.) 'And what is *this*?' She poked her walking stick at the framed bits of paper.

'Um ... well, that's as far as we've got with our research,' admitted Jaz.

'I don't suppose *you* have any ideas about what it could be, Dr Bennet?' said Rosy hopefully.

'Oh, my dears, *I'm* no historian, medical history or otherwise. No, no, English Literature, that's my passion. However, I *can* tell you that those pages must have been printed prior to 1810.'

'Really? How do you know?' said Jaz, snatching up her notebook.

'Is it to do with how yellow the paper is?' said Rosy. 'Or the colour of the ink or –'

'No, it's simply that English printers had stopped using the long "s" form by 1810. Notice the word "scurvy" at the top of the page. That's a long "s" right there.'

'But that's an "f",' protested Jaz. 'It's got a line across its middle.'

'Confusing, isn't it?' said Dr Bennet cheerfully. 'However, that's how they printed the letter "s" prior to the nineteenth century. I believe it was derived from the old Roman cursive form. The long "s" was only used at the beginning or in the middle of a word, of course.' She pointed to the word 'fpoonfuls'. '*Spoonfuls*, you see. And then, down here, what looks like "greedinefs" is *greediness*.'

'This book's about how to cure scurvy!' said Rosy. 'Oranges and lemons – that's what they used to stop scurvy on long sea voyages!'

'But what does scurvy represent?' wondered Jaz. 'In the history of medicine, I mean.'

'Well, I shall leave you girls to continue your research,' said Dr Bennet. 'As for me, I believe it is time for morning tea. I can hear Lynette's delicious caramel slice summoning me down to the office …'

Back in Rosy's room, Rosy and Jaz turned to their preferred sources of wisdom.

'So, we're looking for something written before 1810, about treating scurvy,' said Jaz, scanning the index of her heftiest book.

'But what *is* scurvy, exactly?' said Rosy, tapping at Methuselah's keyboard. 'I know sailors used to get it but – Oh, here it is! A disease caused by a lack of vitamin C, leading to the slow, painful breakdown of the body's connective tissues, including skin, teeth, cartilage, bones and ligaments. Urgh,

Chapter Eleven

look at this disgusting picture of someone's teeth falling out –'

'Listen to this,' interrupted Jaz. 'In 1740, a British naval hero called George Anson set out to circumnavigate the world. When he returned home a few years later, only four of his men had died in battle, but over a *thousand* had died of scurvy! That was more than two-thirds of his crew.'

'No fresh fruit or vegetables on long voyages, so no vitamin C,' said Rosy, nodding. 'Not that they knew about vitamin C then. Or did they?'

'Not at that stage. The navy must have been desperate to find a cure,' said Jaz. 'Oh, here's a British naval surgeon called James Lind who wrote a book called *A Treatise of the Scurvy*.'

'When was that?'

'1753.'

'That could be the one,' said Rosy. 'Remember, our fragment of paper had "of the scurvy" written at the top, with something smudgy before it. I don't suppose there's a picture of the book's pages?'

'Let me see if I can find a scan online.' And Jaz pushed Rosy away from Methuselah, ignoring her protests. 'Then we can read the rest of the chapter and work out why Dr Huxley chose those particular pages for his collection and – Rosy! This university owns an original edition of Lind's book!'

'Really?'

'Here it is in their library catalogue. It's in the Rare Books Collection and that's – Oh, Methuselah!'

'I *told* you to be careful with him. Now look what you've done!'

'The Rare Books Collection,' said Jaz, oblivious to Rosy's frantic attempts to revive Methuselah. 'That's in the basement of the main library. No one's allowed to *borrow* rare books, of course, but you can look at them. That is, if you've got a university library card …' She turned and gazed meaningfully at Rosy.

Ten minutes later, they were barrelling through the doors of the Departments of Biochemistry and Microbiology. Rosy's mum had not been in her flat, but nor was she in her office or her laboratory. Eventually they tracked down her secretary, who informed them that Alison had just left for a meeting in the city.

'She said she'd be back by lunchtime,' said the secretary, rather unhelpfully.

'Thanks,' said Rosy. She and Jaz grimaced at each other after the secretary had turned away, then the two girls slouched back outside.

'Now what?' said Jaz. 'Do we wait around here for a couple of hours or –'

Rosy suddenly straightened up. She pressed her finger to her lips, then pointed at the shadowy area below the walkway, where a familiar figure was leaning against the wall. Jaz raised her eyebrows and inclined her head toward the steps. Rosy nodded. They tiptoed downstairs and round the corner, and were pleased to see that their prey remained unaware of their approach.

'Smoking is really bad for you, you know,' announced Rosy loudly.

Chapter Eleven

Marcus leapt several centimetres into the air and dropped his cigarette into the dust. 'Holy mackerel! What are you *doing*, sneaking up on people like that?'

'Do you know that cigarettes contain more than sixty lethal chemicals?' said Jaz. 'And that each cigarette you smoke greatly increases your risk of lung cancer, heart attacks, strokes, stomach ulcers, blindness, gangrene –'

'But I've given up,' protested Marcus weakly. 'Honestly, this is the first cigarette I've had all year!'

'It's only the second week of January,' Rosy pointed out. 'Your resolve didn't last very long.'

'Well, I'm having a stressful morning,' he said. He picked up his dusty cigarette stub, gave it a tragic look, then squashed it inside the empty cigarette packet he took from the pocket of his jeans. '*Extremely* stressful. The results of our research grant applications are being released today and everyone's on edge. I got so distracted, I dropped a whole tray of Petri dishes this morning. I'm going to have to do them all over again.'

'Then it's a good thing we stopped you finishing that cigarette,' said Jaz. 'Because smoking increases your blood pressure and decreases the amount of oxygen reaching your brain. Imagine how much worse your mental state would be, if *we* hadn't come along.'

'What are you two doing here, anyway?' Marcus squinted at them. 'Dr Radford went into the city to meet with that advisory committee.'

'Yeah, we know that *now*,' said Rosy. 'But that's okay, because you're here. Can we borrow your library card?'

'What, so you can carry out some nefarious scheme and blame it on me? No way, José.'

'It's not nefarious!' said Rosy, even though she wasn't exactly sure what "nefarious" meant. It sounded bad, though. 'Come on, it'll help our investigation.'

'No lending out library cards. Can't be done.'

'Well, come with us to the library, then,' said Rosy. '*Please*. It won't take long. We just need to look at one little book. It's not as though you're doing any work right now, anyway.'

'No, I was having a *relaxing break* until you arrived. Why should I help you lot?'

Rosy and Jaz exchanged a long, thoughtful look.

'What does your mum think about smoking?' Jaz asked Rosy conversationally.

'Oh, she hates it,' replied Rosy. 'She would be extremely disappointed if she heard that one of her students was sneaking out of the lab to poison his lungs when he's actually supposed to be studying Petri dishes. Although, of course, if he came with us to the library, we wouldn't have to mention it to her …'

'Blackmail?' said Marcus. 'Ha! That will never work on me. *Never*.'

'The Mr Gelato van is parked outside the library,' said Rosy. 'We'll buy you an ice-cream.'

'Bribery, on the other hand,' said Marcus, 'is occasionally successful. All right, then. But only because the research grant results won't be posted on their website till twelve o'clock.'

'Yay! Thanks, Marcus!' cried Rosy and Jaz, and they dragged him off to the library, which turned out to be

Chapter Eleven

deserted, apart from half a dozen librarians standing about behind various counters.

'They're probably grateful to have something interesting to do,' whispered Rosy, after Jaz had filled out a request slip and given it to Marcus, who handed it and his library card to one of the librarians. Jaz had already turned back to the computer catalogue, but Rosy's attention was caught by a display of old books in a glass-fronted cabinet. 'Ooh, Jaz, come and look at this! It's a copy of *Malleus Maleficarum*! That'll come in handy if the library is invaded by witches.'

'First edition?' asked Jaz, glancing over.

'No, seventh. Published in 1520.'

'Oh,' said Jaz. 'Hey, Rosy, did you know this library owns two early editions of *De Humani Corporis Fabrica*?'

'Cool. I wish *they* were on display. Those skeleton pictures are awesome. Hmm, what's this book down here? It's by ... Dioscorides. Never heard of him. Nice illustrations, though.'

'Is that *De Materia Medica*? That's about medicinal plants, written by a Greek physician in the first century AD,' said Jaz, going over to join Rosy. 'Highly influential for the next fifteen centuries, although not very accurate –'

The woman sitting behind the desk seemed quite impressed by their knowledge of antiquarian texts. 'Are these girls your students?' she asked Marcus.

'Well, no, they're –'

'Actually, we're supervising his thesis,' Rosy told her.

'He needs a *lot* of supervision,' said Jaz, nodding.

'Oi –!' said Marcus, but he was interrupted by the other librarian, who'd returned with their requested book. She took them into a small reading room, where she seated them at a table and handed Marcus a pair of white cotton gloves, warning him to be very careful when turning each page.

'This is definitely the same book,' said Rosy, leaning over his shoulder. 'Look at the typeface!'

'Oh, and by the way, Marcus,' said Jaz, at his other shoulder, 'if you see something that looks like a lower-case "f" and it's not at the end of a word, it's probably an "s".'

'Okay,' said Marcus, examining the title page. 'And why exactly are we interested in *A Treatise of the Scurvy. In Three Parts. Containing An inquiry into the Nature, Causes and Cure, of that Disease. By James Lind, M.D.*?'

'We don't know yet. That's what we're trying to find out,' said Rosy.

'Turn to Chapter Four,' said Jaz. 'Keep going ... There, that's it! No, go back a page. Rosy, look at this: "I took twelve patients in the scurvy ... Their cases were as similar as I could have them ... They lay together in one place ... and had one diet common to all." And then he divided the men into six pairs and gave each pair a different treatment for scurvy.'

'He's using the scientific method!' said Rosy. 'The first medical treatment trial in history! Do you think? Oh, no, wait, there was that French surgeon, wasn't there, centuries before? The one who ran out of boiling oil to pour on the soldiers' wounds, so half his patients got rose ointment instead, and then he compared the two groups to see which healed better.'

'But Ambroise Paré didn't design his trial carefully and then carry it out,' said Jaz. 'He couldn't, because he was in the middle of a battlefield. He probably treated the most severely wounded soldiers first – at least, that's what I'd have done – so the worst wounds would have been treated with boiling oil, not ointment. Maybe it wasn't the *treatment* that made the difference. Maybe the wounds themselves were different. James Lind is doing something new here – he's starting off by making sure all the patients are the same, so he can do a fair comparison.'

'Randomly assigning patients to treatment groups,' said Marcus, nodding. 'As well as controlling for variables.'

'Wait, what did you say?' asked Rosy. 'Controlling for *variables*? That was the bit I didn't understand when Mum was explaining about the scientific method.'

'It means making sure that the only thing in the experiment that varies is the medical treatment,' said Marcus. 'See, these scurvy patients had the same disease, with symptoms of about the same severity, were kept in the same place and ate the same food … And it says they're all sailors on the same ship, so they're all men and probably all about the same age. The only thing that's different is the treatment they receive. One treatment group gets cider; one gets "elixir vitriol", which I think is diluted sulphuric acid; one gets vinegar; one gets sea water; one gets a mixture of garlic, mustard and whatever "rad. raphan" and "balsam of Peru" are; and the last group gets two oranges and a lemon each day.

'Plus, he has another group that had no treatment at all. That's the control group, to see if the disease gets better by itself. At the end of the trial, if any treatment group shows significantly more improvement than the control group, that treatment must have had a real effect.'

'Oh, that makes sense,' said Rosy. 'Man, I bet all those sailors wished they'd been in the oranges-and-lemons group! Imagine being in the group that had to drink half a pint of sea water a day.'

'Especially as the men who had the citrus fruit were the only ones who showed "sudden and visible good effects",' said Jaz, pointing at the page. 'Look, one of those sailors was back at work in six days and the other was well enough to act as a nurse for the other patients. It's pretty clear which treatment worked the best.'

'And Lind even included a review of all the previous literature on scurvy treatments,' observed Marcus, turning back to an earlier section. 'Just like we medical researchers have to do these days.' He looked over his shoulder at Jaz, who'd been busily taking notes. 'But you don't need to read all that, do you?'

'Well ...' said Jaz.

'Jaz, it's four hundred and fifty-six pages long,' said Rosy. 'We can't make poor Marcus go through the whole book. Anyway, now we know why Dr Huxley chose those pages. This object is about nutrition!

Chapter Eleven

The importance of vitamins! How a balanced diet is essential for good health!'

'What? No, it's not,' said Jaz. 'It's about designing effective medical research!'

Marcus took advantage of the ensuing argument to summon the librarian. 'So, can we go now?' he asked the girls, after the librarian had collected the book and handed him back his library card.

'Just a couple more minutes,' said Jaz, grabbing his card. 'I need to find out how long it took for the navy to act on these results.' Then she dashed down the corridor. Marcus sighed, but trailed uncomplainingly after Rosy to the main room, where Jaz had logged on to a computer and was now examining a site dedicated to James Lind. 'His results were so clear,' she announced indignantly when they arrived at her side, 'but look, they ignored his evidence for decades!'

'It was a pretty small trial, though,' said Marcus. 'Only twelve experimental subjects. And it's not as though they had medical journals or internet forums to spread the news in those days.'

'Actually, it *was* sort of Lind's fault,' conceded Jaz, scrolling down the page. 'It says here he took years to write up his research and then his recommended scurvy treatment was a concentrated form of lemon juice, which he thought would be easier to store on ships. But boiling the lemon juice to evaporate it destroyed all its vitamin C, so it didn't help with scurvy at all and most people lost interest. It wasn't till 1780 that Gilbert Blane read Lind's work and set up his own much bigger trial. And even then, it took till 1795 before the British Admiralty ordered all its sailors to be issued with lemon juice rations.'

'Hey, but what about James Cook?' said Rosy. 'The *Endeavour* sailed around the world for years and none of the crew died of scurvy. And remember, he landed in Australia in 1770. That's decades before official lemon rations.'

'Let me check,' said Jaz, turning back to the keyboard. 'Hmm ... Cook was definitely ahead of his time. It says he believed a varied diet prevented scurvy, so he made sure there was lots of pickled cabbage and fresh greens and citrus fruit available. The crew weren't very keen on the pickled cabbage and refused to eat it, so Cook had it served only to the officers, making it seem like some sort of delicacy, and then everyone wanted some.'

'Clever,' said Rosy. 'So, if it weren't for Cook and his sneaky scurvy-preventing cabbage, the British wouldn't have made it to Botany Bay. And they wouldn't have been the first Europeans to set up a colony here and we'd probably all be speaking French now instead. Of course, *I* can speak it anyway ...'

'No, you can't,' said Jaz. 'Not properly. Oh, this is a bit sad. James Lind died just before the Admiralty gave the order about lemon juice rations, so he never knew that they'd finally taken his advice.'

'Taken it on board, so to speak,' said Marcus.

'What's that?' Rosy leaned over and pointed at a heading. '*The Strange Disappearances of James Lind.*'

'It seems his body vanished after his funeral,' said Jaz, scanning the article.

Chapter Eleven

'Body-snatchers!'

'No –'

'He turned into a zombie?'

Marcus started laughing. 'Shh,' Jaz hissed at him. 'This *is* a library, you know.' Which only made Marcus laugh even louder. Jaz shook her head disapprovingly and turned back to the computer. 'No, it's just that they couldn't find Lind's body when they opened his vault in Portchester Castle church. It was missing for centuries, but then a few years ago, someone saw a slab in the castle grounds with his name on it, so he's probably buried there. I bet they just recorded it wrongly in the first place.'

'Well, that's a boring story,' said Rosy. 'Zombies would have been a lot more interesting.'

'Speaking of zombies,' Jaz said, 'this computer is a lot faster than Methuselah. Like, about a hundred times faster.'

'All right, all right, he does his best,' said Rosy. 'Let's see how fast *you* are when you're a thousand years old. But while you're here, look up when vitamin C was discovered. And who figured out the whole idea of vitamin deficiencies.'

'Look up Dumas,' suggested Marcus, whose laughter had subsided, somewhat. 'And Lunin.'

Jaz gave him a suspicious glance, but it turned out to be good advice. 'Write this down, Rosy,' she ordered. 'Jean-Baptiste Dumas was looking after starving babies during the 1871 siege of Paris when he ran out of milk. He tried feeding them a mixture of fat, sugar and protein, but he found that wasn't enough to nourish them. And then Nikolai Ivanovich Lunin fed rats synthetic milk made of fat, protein, carbohydrates and salts, but the rats *still* died. So there had to be something extra in food that made it nutritious and helped animals grow.

'In 1912, Frederick Gowland Hopkins worked out that these "accessory food factors" existed in tiny quantities. Then Casimir Funk actually isolated one of these substances from rice husks. He named them "vital amines" or "vitamines". And *then* scientists started discovering lots of different vitamins. Vitamin A in butter, vitamin B in eggs and yeast, vitamin D in cod-liver oil, vitamin E in green leafy vegetables –'

'And vitamin C?' asked Rosy.

'Albert Szent-Györgyi won the Nobel Prize in 1937 for isolating vitamin C and making a synthetic version.'

Rosy nodded. 'Good work, Albert. Although Casimir Funk won the award for having the coolest name.'

'And then they figured out which diseases were caused by vitamin deficiencies. Like, rickets is caused by lack of vitamin D. Oh, *this* is interesting –'

'Aren't you done yet?' said Marcus plaintively.

'You sound like my little brother,' Rosy told him. 'And he's three. *Are we there yet? Can we go now?*'

'*I want my ice-cream!*' squeaked Marcus.

'Okay, okay, hang on, I'll just print out these pages,' said Jaz.

Then they went outside to the ice-cream van, which was parked in a shady corner of the courtyard. Marcus chose Pistachio and Rum-Raisin, because

Chapter Eleven

he was working his way through the thirty-seven available flavours in alphabetical order. Rosy had Chocolate Swirl and Double Choc-Chip with chocolate sprinkles on top and Jaz, who took ice-cream decisions as seriously as she did everything else, eventually decided on Pineapple and Lime.

'Staving off scurvy?' Marcus asked her, as they sat down under the tree with their already-melting ice-creams.

'I doubt there's much vitamin C in this,' said Jaz. 'I'm not sure it has any nutritional value at all. It tastes pretty good, though.'

'It's got calcium in it, hasn't it?' said Rosy. 'And don't dairy foods have vitamins added to them?'

'Oh, that reminds me,' said Jaz, pulling out her notebook one-handed. 'Did you know that it's impossible to get enough vitamin D from food, even if you eat heaps of eggs and fish and dairy products? You need exposure to sunlight as well, because UV rays make vitamin D when they hit your skin. But scientists did some research a few years ago and found that even in summer, one in three Sydney office workers have a vitamin D deficiency. That causes bone diseases – and maybe even depression and heart disease and cancer.'

'So – what?' said Rosy. 'We're all supposed to sit outside and get burnt to a crisp? What happened to "Slip, Slop, Slap"?'

'Well, that's the problem,' said Jaz. 'Too much sun causes skin cancer, especially in Australia. Two thousand people die of it here each year. But not *enough* sun can make people sick, too. And anyway, each person needs a different amount of sun, depending on where they live and their medical history and all sorts of other things. Like, my skin's darker than yours, so I'd need more time in the sun to make the same amount of vitamin D. Scientists can't even agree about how much vitamin D we need to be healthy. In North America, the official recommended amount is three times as much as in Australia.'

'Well, if *scientists* don't know, how are we supposed to?' said Rosy.

'They just need to do more research,' said Marcus, popping the end of his ice-cream cone into his mouth. 'There ought to be more funding for medical scientists. Especially brilliant, hard-working, post-grad microbiology students. Speaking of which …' He stood up and brushed some crumbs off his T-shirt, which read: 'HAVE NO FEAR: THE MICROBIOLOGIST IS HERE'.

'Do you have an entire wardrobe of those shirts?' said Rosy. 'Where do you get them from?'

'People keep giving me them for birthdays and Christmas. I think they order them online. Anyway, I'd better get back to saving humankind from the menace of infectious diseases.'

'Thanks for the library card,' said Jaz.

'And good luck with the research grant,' said Rosy.

'Cheers. See you later, Thomson and Thompson.'

He waved goodbye and strode off.

'Who's … Hang on!' said Rosy. 'Those bumbling detectives in *Tintin*? We're nothing like them!'

But Jaz's mind was elsewhere. 'Maybe you're right,' she said, as they stood up and headed back to

Chapter Eleven

New College. 'I mean, about this object being related to nutrition. Maybe Dr Huxley wanted to show that improving health isn't just about killing bacteria or doing effective surgery, that it's also about things like adding vitamins to food and not eating too much salt.'

'Yeah,' said Rosy. 'Except they keep changing their minds about that. Like, first, fat was the most evil thing in the world, except then they decided some types of fats were good, and then it was carbohydrates that were out, and now it's sugar, so that even fruit juice is bad for you and –'

'I don't think it's scientists saying those things. I think it's the people who write about diets in magazines. Although at least they're trying to give us information about health.'

'Maybe there's such a thing as *too much* information,' said Rosy. 'We've got tonnes of facts about food and exercise now, but I watched this thing on TV that said our generation might be the first in history to live *shorter* lives than our parents and grandparents, because we've got such high rates of diabetes and heart disease. Which is probably because we're sitting around watching TV and eating chocolate ice-creams …'

'There's nothing wrong with watching TV or eating an occasional ice-cream, it's when you … EEP!' Jaz grabbed Rosy's arm and yanked them both into the shadows of the cloisters.

'When you *eep*?' said Rosy. 'What are you on about?'

'Shh!' said Jaz, peeking round a sandstone pillar. 'It's Ms Boydell! What's she doing here? Do you think she's following us?'

Rosy peered over Jaz's shoulder. A slim dark-haired figure in a navy suit paused on the flagstone path, gazed around the quadrangle, then continued tip-tapping along in her stiletto heels. 'Well … she *could* be,' said Rosy. 'Or she could just be getting some parking permits for the conference visitors next week.'

'Oh,' said Jaz, as Ms Boydell disappeared inside a doorway marked "ADMINISTRATION". 'I forgot about that. Dad's meant to have finished all the landscaping around the front path by then. What sort of conference is it, anyway?'

Rosy shrugged. 'Dunno. It's only two days. We're meant to stay out of the refectory, though, because they're having a fancy dinner in there on Monday night.'

Jaz was frowning. 'Ms Boydell still hasn't asked Dad to do a quote for landscaping all of the college grounds. Maybe she knows what we did. Maybe she knows the college won't end up getting the money from Dr Huxley's estate after all. Maybe – Why are we going this way?'

'I just need to check something about my Midnight Visitor,' said Rosy. 'You wait here. I won't be long.' Ignoring Jaz's protests, she tugged open the door of the Macleay Museum and raced upstairs, clattering back down a few minutes later.

'Well?' said Jaz, eyebrows raised and arms crossed. Rosy shook her head ruefully.

'"The great tragedy of Science – the slaying of a beautiful hypothesis by an ugly fact."'

'Who said that?' asked Jaz.

Chapter Eleven

'I did,' said Rosy. 'Just then.'

'No, I mean, who said it originally?'

'Oh, Huxley. Not ours, the other one.'

They crossed the road and headed downhill.

'But it's not all bad,' Rosy added, 'because I did discover a fact that might turn out to be even *more* useful.'

'Which you're not going to tell me.'

'No, not yet,' said Rosy. 'I need to plan my experiment first.'

'Fine,' said Jaz. 'Be all mysterious. But don't forget our priority is figuring out Dr Huxley's next object. And you know what that is?'

Rosy thought for a moment, then groaned. 'Oh no! Not –'

'The creepy head,' said Jaz, nodding.

CHAPTER TWELVE

'... now, when science is strong and religion weak, men mistake medicine for magic.'
~ Thomas Szasz

The creepy head had not become any less creepy in the four days Rosy had spent avoiding its gaze.

'As if those staring eyes weren't bad enough,' she complained, 'there's that horrible gaping hole in its throat!'

'Maybe it's some sort of practice head for medical students,' said Jaz. 'You know how sometimes patients stop breathing, so the doctors put a tube in their throat to give them oxygen? Maybe students used this to learn how to insert the tube.' She lifted the porcelain head, which was about half the size of a real one, and peered down the hole. 'It's hollow inside. And painted black. No, dark blue.'

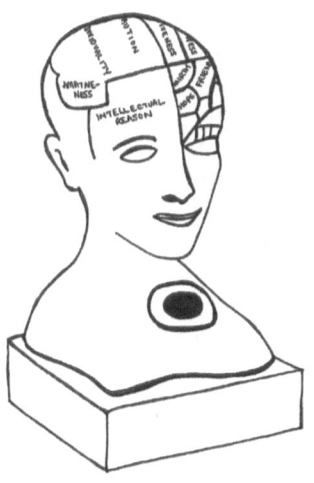

'Painted? What, *inside*? Why would they do that?

~ 185 ~

And what about these words written all over it? *Inhabitiveness. Concentrativeness.* Look at this one – *Philoprogenitiveness*! What does that even mean?'

'You said that something about it seemed familiar,' said Jaz, replacing the head on its shelf, 'when we first saw it.'

'Yeah,' said Rosy. 'It did. It does. I've just got this ... feeling.' She glanced warily at Jaz, but Jaz only nodded. Perhaps she was remembering how Rosy's intuition had led them up the museum stairs to Pasteur's flask. Rosy continued with more confidence. 'You see, for some reason, it makes me think of my dad. But I don't know why.'

'Could he have owned one of these, ages ago?'

'No, I don't think so.' Rosy furrowed her brow, but the feeling, strong as it was, didn't seem to be connected to a clear thought. It was very frustrating. The memory was lurking in her brain, hiding just out of reach ...

'Hey, Jaz,' she said. 'What's a memory? What's a thought? Is it a *thing*? I mean, I'm thinking now, but what's going on in my brain? Or in your brain? Anyone's brain?'

'Well, there are cells in the brain, nerve cells,' said Jaz, 'and they send electrical signals to each other using chemicals called, um ... neurotransmitters. I think that's right. I don't think a thought is a *thing*, exactly. It's like, if you have a car and you've put petrol in the tank and you turn the key, you'll get movement and speed, but that speed only exists sometimes, when the

Chapter Twelve

car's working. Speed is something that happens due to the car, like a thought happens in a brain.'

'Hmm,' said Rosy, pondering this. 'Chemicals and electricity. I'm thinking really, *really* hard right now. Do you reckon if I do it too long, my head will explode?'

'I doubt it,' said Jaz. 'Just concentrate on the head, will you? The creepy head, not yours.'

Rosy squeezed her eyes shut. Could she have seen a head like this at an art exhibition? One that her dad had taken her to? No, that wasn't it ...

'Marcus,' she said, opening her eyes suddenly. 'It's something to do with Marcus, as well.'

'Marcus?' said Jaz. 'Marcus and your dad? Okay. They're both ... male. What else? Learning. University? Research?'

'No, but keep going – this is great. Word associations! Dad says they're good for unlocking the mind. Brain. Whatever.'

'Um, Petri dishes? Bacteria? Honey?'

'No ...'

'Ice-cream? Sherlock? Ninjas?'

'T-shirts!' cried Rosy. 'It was on Dad's old T-shirt! He wore it all the time and it got so full of holes that Gabrielle made him cut it up for paint rags. It had a picture on it of this sort of head, with writing all over the skull. Oh, man, I wish he was somewhere with mobile coverage so I could ring him and ask, but they don't even have proper internet up there.'

'Would your mum know?'

'Maybe. She should be back by now, shouldn't she?'

They raced down to the flat, where Alison was unpacking some groceries.

'Mum! Mum! Remember that old T-shirt of Dad's, with the head that had writing all over it? What was it? What did it mean?'

Alison shut the fridge door. 'You mean his REMO shirt? The one I gave him for his birthday?'

'What's a Remo?' demanded Rosy, as Jaz whipped out her notebook and pen. 'What does it do?'

'It sells things,' said Alison. 'It's a shop. Or it was – I think the shop closed down and they moved online. Why?'

'A shop!' Rosy collapsed on the sofa. 'No, I meant that head picture with the writing on it!'

'Oh, that's the shop's logo. A phrenology head. I guess they thought it was all retro and cool.'

'Is *phrenology* spelled with a "ph" or an "f"?' said Jaz. 'Hmm, probably a "ph" …'

'But what *is* phrenology?' said Rosy.

'A bit of Victorian pseudoscience,' said Alison, picking up her keys. 'Now, Rosy, listen. I have to go back to the lab for a little while, but then –'

'Yeah, okay, fine,' said Rosy, already looking about for Methuselah. 'Oh, wait!' she added, as Alison reached the door. 'Did Marcus get his research grant?'

'Yes, of course he did,' said Alison. 'It was a brilliant application and it's exactly the sort of practical, clever research that – Hang on, you haven't been bothering him while he's working, have you?'

'No,' said Rosy, which was true. (He *hadn't* been doing any work that morning.)

Chapter Twelve

'I sincerely hope not –' began Alison sternly, but then her phone rang and she rushed off, stuffing photocopies in her bag and scattering paper clips over the carpet.

'Right, phrenology,' said Jaz, after they'd located Methuselah and coaxed him back into life. 'Are you taking notes? Okay, so around 1800, Franz Joseph Gall came up with this idea that the brain was made up of twenty-seven individual organs connected to a person's character and abilities. There was a brain organ for language, and one for musical talent, and another for understanding colours. But there were also organs for vanity, cunning, arrogance – even theft and murder. He thought the more a person used a particular organ, the bigger it would get, so there'd be a bump on the skull in a specific place to show this. He spent years measuring skulls and matching them to people's personalities and skills.'

'So that's what the writing on the creepy head is!' said Rosy. 'It's a head map with labels.'

'Right. Then Gall's assistant, Johann Spurzheim, published his *Physiognomical System* in 1815, making the labels more specific and Thomas Forster introduced the name *phrenology*, meaning "the study of the mind". But it was the Fowler brothers, Orson and Lorenzo, who made it really popular, selling pamphlets and charts and ceramic phrenology heads to the public. Plus, there were phrenology snuffboxes, phrenology cane handles, phrenology … inkwells! That's what Dr Huxley's head is! I mean, not *his* head, but –'

'Ours looks just like the one in that photo,' said Rosy, pointing at the screen. '"An antique phrenology inkwell, circa 1850." *That's* why it's dark blue inside — it used to have ink in it.'

'It says here Mark Twain got his head read by Lorenzo Fowler,' said Jaz, 'and what Fowler told him about his character was totally wrong. Then Twain went back three months later giving a different name and he got a completely different analysis of his character and it was *still* wrong.'

'Ha!'

'Some people seemed to take it very seriously, though. They used phrenology to decide whether to employ someone or who they should marry. Or even whether someone was a criminal or not. That was really popular in Australia, maybe because there were so many convicts here. Phrenologists used to make plaster casts of bushrangers' skulls to analyse them. See, here's one of Captain Moonlite —'

'And Ned Kelly!' said Rosy, who'd forgotten she was supposed to be taking notes. 'Let's see what the phrenologist had to say about him! Okay, according to A. S. Hamilton, "travelling phrenologist", Ned Kelly had huge organs of destructiveness and combativeness and ambition, and tiny organs of cautiousness and conscientiousness.'

'Wow, amazing,' said Jaz, very sarcastically. 'I wonder how the phrenologist reached that conclusion. Possibly because he was examining the skull of Australia's most notorious criminal, who'd just been hanged for robbing banks and murdering all those policemen?'

'Well, yeah, but phrenologists studied the skulls of people who weren't criminals, too. Look at these two

Chapter Twelve

phrenologists who stole the head of Joseph Haydn, the composer, from his grave and found that his skull's bump of music was –'

'Let me guess, it was *gigantic*,' said Jaz. 'Honestly, this is ridiculous. It's so … unscientific!'

'No, it's not,' protested Rosy. 'There *are* different bits of the brain that do different things. Like, when my grandpa had his stroke, the doctors did all these scans of his brain and found exactly where the damaged bits were and they said, "Oh, his right arm and leg will be weak and he'll have problems saying sentences, but he'll understand what you say." And that's exactly what happened, and he had to have loads of physiotherapy and speech therapy, and he got better. Well, a bit better. He still needs a walking frame to get around.'

'That's different. Of course there are specific areas of your brain doing specific things, but that has nothing to do with how the outside of your skull looks.'

'But the *idea* behind it was good,' said Rosy. 'It's just that they didn't have brain scanning machines then, so it was hard to prove … Oh, hi, Mum. That was quick.'

'Forgot my backup drive,' said Alison, rummaging through the papers on her desk.

'You don't *need* brain scanning machines to work things out scientifically,' said Jaz. 'Here, look at David Ferrier. He was studying epilepsy in the 1870s and he figured out which parts of the brain caused certain muscles to move or stop moving by, er …'

'Oh, by doing horrible experiments on poor little rabbits and dogs and monkeys! Cutting out bits of their brains and giving them electric shocks to find out how they reacted!'

'I know it's horrible,' said Jaz, 'but how else was he supposed to learn?'

'Actually, his main problem was that dog and monkey brains are different to human brains,' said Alison, peering over their shoulders. 'So his results were inaccurate. But there *was* another method. Look up Broca.'

'Okay,' said Rosy, after she'd established that Paul Broca spelled his name with a 'c' rather than a 'k'. 'So, Broca found people in hospital who'd stopped being able to talk, waited till they died, then cut open their brains to find out where the damaged parts were. Clever.'

'And look, so did Carl Wernicke,' said Jaz. 'He discovered the part of the brain that helps us understand speech and that's why it's called Wernicke's area.'

'Oh, there's a Broca's area, too, that helps us talk. Well, this is *much* better than experimenting on animals,' Rosy said. 'Although sometimes it must have been a bit frustrating for the scientists. What if they found someone with a fascinating disorder, but then the person stayed alive for years and years?'

'Someone like Phineas Gage,' said Alison.

Rosy and Jaz lunged for Methuselah's keyboard. Rosy got there first. 'Urgh!' She reeled back almost immediately. 'Why did I click on the article with the pictures?'

'How did he manage to survive that accident at *all*, let alone live for twelve years?' marvelled Jaz. 'A

Chapter Twelve

crowbar got propelled right through his head! Look at the hole in his skull!'

'It says his personality changed completely,' said Rosy. 'He turned stubborn and impatient and he wouldn't stop swearing. See, phrenology wasn't totally wrong. Phrenologists *said* that would happen if you damaged your organs of benevolence and veneration.'

'Except those organs are supposed to be in the middle of the skull and Gage's brain damage was on the left,' pointed out Jaz. 'Anyway, his personality couldn't have been *that* badly affected, if he got a job as a coach driver afterwards. I bet phrenologists just made up stuff about him to fit their theories. Look, they claimed he abused his wife and children, and he didn't even *have* a wife or children. Phrenology's not science. It's people *pretending* to do science.'

'Oh, well,' said Rosy. 'Phineas Gage had his accident back in the 1840s. People didn't know as much about science then. They wouldn't say those sorts of things now.'

Alison snorted. 'Don't bet on it. There's plenty of pseudoscience around today. What about chiropractic? What about *homeopathy*?'

'Oh, Mum,' groaned Rosy, grabbing a cushion and squashing it over her ears. 'Don't start on that again.'

'All right. I'm going now,' said Alison. '*Homeopathy*,' she mouthed in Jaz's direction, before disappearing out the door.

Jaz turned to Rosy enquiringly.

'You don't want to know,' said Rosy, rolling her eyes. 'Let's just say that Gabrielle has this homeopath friend who happened to drop off a remedy for Reuben's earache one day when Mum was visiting, and it turned into World War Three in our kitchen.'

'Oh,' said Jaz. 'Right. So … it's some sort of alternative medicine, is it? I've never heard of it before.'

Rosy slumped down further on the sofa. 'Okay.' She shoved the cushion under her head. 'Here's what I know and I consider myself an expert on the subject after listening to all the arguing that day. There was this German doctor, Samuel Hahnemann, right, about two hundred years ago, and he thought diseases – or at least, symptoms of diseases – were caused by the body's vital force getting disturbed. And he also noticed that when he took this particular malaria medicine made out of powdered bark, it made him – a healthy person – feel all feverish and thirsty, as though he really *did* have malaria. Mum said it was probably only because he happened to be allergic to it, but anyway, he decided that if a substance causes symptoms in healthy people, you can use that substance to treat the same symptoms in sick people. So he did a lot of what he called "provings", where he gave people different substances and recorded exactly how they felt while they were taking them, so he could work out what the substances cured.'

Jaz was wearing a very familiar look, which indicated she was about to launch into a flurry of questions, but Rosy pressed on.

'Oh, and I forgot to say some of the substances were really poisonous, so he started diluting them using this special procedure he invented, where he added one drop in a flask to a hundred drops of water and banged the flask ten times against a board, and then he kept diluting that solution again and again. He also said that the more dilute the solution was, the more powerful it became. And that's what homeopathic medicine is. You go to a homeopath and they ask lots of questions about your symptoms, your medical history, your lifestyle and all that, then they match your information to their reference books and give you some homeopathic medicine. So, for instance, coffee makes most people more alert and awake, so if someone feels irritable and can't sleep, they might be prescribed a remedy based on coffee.'

'That ... doesn't make a lot of sense.' Jaz was frowning. 'And how many dilutions did you say they do for each medicine?'

'It depends. I think lots of them are diluted thirty times, but some are diluted a hundred or even two hundred times.'

'Thirty,' mused Jaz. 'So that's one in one hundred to the power of thirty, which means ten to the power of sixty ...'

'Are you doing maths? Please stop that. I'm allergic to maths.'

'You are not allergic to maths. Listen. A million is a one with six zeros after it, okay? It's a very big number. Well, imagine a one with *sixty* zeros after it. That is an enormous number of drops of water, probably more water than there is on the whole planet. Now add just

Dr Huxley's Bequest

one drop of whatever the medicine substance is and mix it in with all that water. Then take a bottle and dip it into the solution. That's what a thirty-times dilution would be. There is almost no chance that a single molecule of the substance would be in the bottle. So homeopathic medicines are just plain water.'

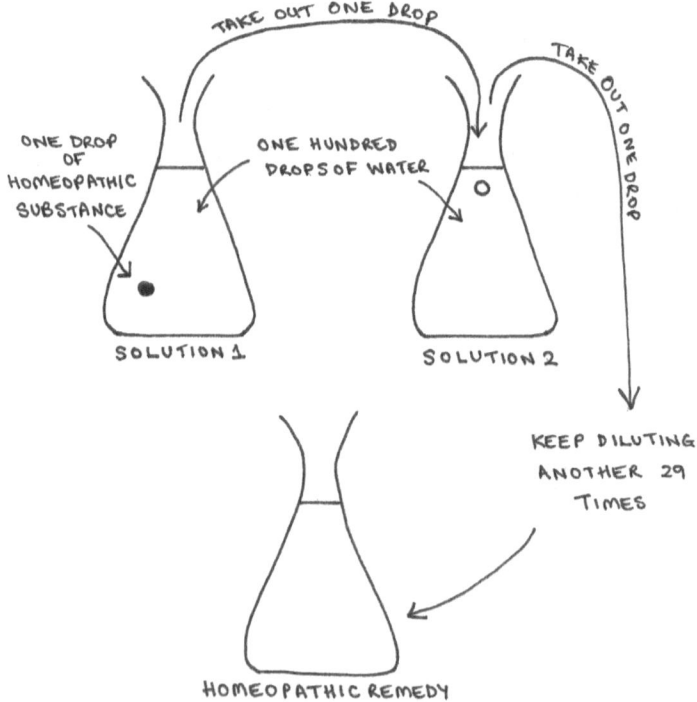

HOMEOPATHIC REMEDY

EQUIVALENT TO ONE DROP OF HOMEOPATHIC SUBSTANCE IN 1, 000, 000, 000, 000, 000, 000, 000, 000, 000, 000, 000, 000, 000, 000, 000, 000, 000, 000, 000 DROPS OF WATER

Chapter Twelve

'Um, yeah, but the thing is, homeopaths say that the water has a *memory* of being near the substance, so the medicine will still work –'

'A memory? What, somehow a water molecule *remembers* that particular substance, but it forgets all the other things it's touched since it came into existence? It's probably touched all sorts of disgusting things!'

'Look, *I* don't know how it works,' said Rosy. 'But Gabrielle reckons it does. She says when she's stressed out and has a headache, she takes this homeopathic remedy and soon she's feeling much better. And her friend Cheryl, the homeopath, said there's evidence it really does work. Like, there was a big cholera epidemic in the 1850s and when they compared the death rates at the London Homeopathic Hospital with some other regular hospital, they found that patients were twice as likely to die in the regular hospital.'

'So what?' said Jaz. 'Regular medical treatment was useless back then. All they had was bloodletting and awful potions full of mercury and arsenic. Patients would have been a lot better off doing something useless but harmless, like taking homeopathic medicine. Anyway, that's not a randomised trial. Maybe there was something different about the patients in each hospital. Maybe the homeopathy hospital was more expensive, so poor patients who were sicker went to the regular hospital. Maybe –'

'Well, that cholera thing was just an example. Apparently there's modern evidence, too.'

Jaz had already seized Methuselah and was typing away. 'Aha!' she said presently. '*The Lancet*, which is a very important medical journal, says that five different groups of scientists analysed all the modern research into homeopathy and concluded that homeopathy has absolutely no medical effect. Well, no more than a placebo, which does have *some* effect on some medical conditions.'

'What's a placebo?'

'A pill with no medicine in it.'

'How could *that* have any effect on a patient?'

'It does if the patient is told that it's actually medicine. No, seriously, there's all sorts of research to prove the placebo effect. It's really interesting. Let's see if I can find … Oh, here it is. Scientists discovered that placebo pills in fancy packets were better at stopping headaches than placebo pills in plain packets. And expensive placebo pills worked better than cheap placebo pills. And placebo pills given by a doctor wearing a white coat were more effective than the same placebo pills given by a nurse.

'They even did an experiment that showed that the *colour* of the placebo pill makes a difference, so for example, blue placebo pills have a more calming effect than pink ones. And it's not just placebo *pills* they've tested. They found placebo injections work better than placebo pills. They've even tested placebo ultrasound treatments and placebo surgery and found that they work better than no treatment at all, as long as the patients believe they're getting real medical treatments.'

'So, what are you saying?' asked Rosy. 'That Gabrielle's headache goes away after taking a

Chapter Twelve

homeopathic remedy because of the placebo effect? Well, does it matter? She still feels better after she takes it.'

'Yes, but aspirin would be a lot more effective. And I bet a packet of aspirin is cheaper than going to see a homeopath.'

'But she *likes* going to see Cheryl. She says Cheryl really listens to her and gives useful advice. And drugs – even aspirin – have side effects. Homeopathic remedies don't.'

Jaz made a huffing noise. 'That's because there's nothing in them but water! And what if people start thinking homeopaths can cure anything, even serious diseases? What if someone gets really sick and refuses to see a proper doctor?'

'Yeah, that's what Mum and Cheryl were arguing about. Because Mum said Reuben needed to see a doctor about his ear infection and Cheryl reckoned he just needed homeopathic medicine to build up his immune system.'

'What did your dad say?'

'He said they were both making *his* ears hurt and he went and locked himself in his studio. But the next day, he and Gabrielle took Reuben to the doctor, which they were going to do anyway, and the doctor gave Reuben some medicine and he stopped crying and rubbing his ears. Gabrielle reckons his ears are still a bit clogged up, though, because he keeps saying "What?" when you talk to him. See, so regular medicine doesn't always work perfectly, either.'

~ 199 ~

'I never claimed it did,' said Jaz. 'But what was that other thing your mum mentioned? Chiropractic? That's for fixing bad backs, isn't it?'

'Oh, yeah. They manipulate your spine or something. But I don't know why she said that was a pseudoscience. It sounds fairly sensible to me.'

'Hmm,' said Jaz, after further typing. 'Well, except for the bit where its founder, Daniel David Palmer, claimed that nearly all diseases were caused by the bones in the spine being misaligned. Oh, and he didn't believe in germ theory, either.'

'When was this?'

'He came up with the idea of chiropractic in 1895, after he supposedly cured a man's deafness by adjusting the man's spine.'

'Well, lots of qualified medical doctors still believed in ridiculous things like bloodletting back then. So what? Doctors are completely different now and chiropractors probably are, too.'

'Except lots of modern chiropractors claim they can cure bed wetting, asthma, allergies, ear infections and learning difficulties just by pushing around the bones in someone's spine, even though there's no evidence it works. And some of them reckon vaccines are useless for preventing infectious diseases.'

Rosy sighed. 'Is there any proof that chiropractic actually fixes bad backs?'

Jaz's fingers flew over the keyboard. 'Scientific research has shown that chiropractic is as effective at treating back pain as physiotherapy, drugs and exercise,

Chapter Twelve

but none of them are very effective and chiropractic is the most expensive,' she said. 'Also, chiropractors tend to recommend lots of spinal X-rays, which don't actually show anything useful and expose patients to a lot of unnecessary radiation, which increases their risk of cancer. Plus, many chiropractic patients experience pain or dizziness due to their treatment. Manipulating the bones in the neck is especially dangerous, because it can damage blood vessels, forming blood clots that travel up to the brain and cause strokes –'

'Okay, okay.' Rosy held up both hands in surrender. 'I just thought chiropractic sounded more scientific than most of the stuff they do at that Healing Centre where Cheryl works. I mean, compared to crystal therapy, Bach flower remedies, reiki –'

'What's reiki?'

'It's a type of massage, where the healer channels her energy into the patient to restore the natural balance.'

'Is that like Therapeutic Touch?' asked Jaz, frowning at Methuselah. 'That's where the healer feels the "human energy field" above the patient's skin to diagnose the illness and then rebalances the energy so it flows properly.'

'Sounds similar,' said Rosy. 'What are you reading?'

'A girl called Emily Rosa designed a scientific study to see whether Therapeutic Touch really worked,' said Jaz, wearing an expression made up of equal parts admiration and resentment. 'Her research was so good that it got published in *The Journal of the American*

Medical Association. In fact, she's the youngest person ever to have a research paper published in a proper medical journal. And she was *nine years old*.'

'Wow,' said Rosy. 'So, too late for us to break that world record, huh?'

'Although her parents did all the mathematical analysis of the results and they reviewed all the previous scientific papers on the subject for her, so it's not like she did it completely by herself. Oh, here's the research paper.' Jaz examined it for a moment. 'Hmm. Actually, this is a really well-designed scientific study …'

'Go on, then. What did she do?'

'Well, the Therapeutic Touch people claim they can feel this "human energy field" by hovering their hands over the patient's skin. If they can't actually feel it, their therapy can't possibly work. So Emily got a whole lot of TT healers and sat them at a table, one at a time, with their hands stretched out through a hole in a dark screen so they couldn't see Emily on the other side. Then Emily flipped a coin to determine whether she'd hover her hand over the healer's right or left hand. The healer had to say which hand was feeling Emily's energy field.'

'And what was the hypothesis?' asked Rosy.

'If TT really works, the healers should say the correct hand one hundred per cent of the time. If the whole idea of human energy fields is rubbish, the healers should get it right about fifty per cent of the time, which is the same as guessing at random. Emily decided eighty per cent correct would be good enough

Chapter Twelve

to prove the healers were actually detecting an energy field. The healers agreed beforehand with Emily's method of testing.'

'Okay. Results?'

'She did two sets of tests. In the first, there were fifteen healers, who got only forty-seven per cent correct. Then she retested seven of the healers, along with six other healers, and they got forty-one per cent correct.'

'So the conclusion is that Therapeutic Touch and the whole idea of human energy fields is a load of rubbish. Well done, Emily! Did she win the Nobel Prize?'

'No, of course not,' said Jaz. 'Although she did win the James Randi Award for Skeptic of the Year.'

'Cool,' said Rosy. 'I wonder why I've never heard of her before? I mean, she should be at *least* as famous as kids who are models or actors.'

'Yeah, she should be.' Jaz shrugged. 'But what *I* want to know is, why do people pay good money to Therapeutic Touch healers and homeopaths and all that, when there's no evidence the treatment works and most of their ideas don't even make sense?'

'Well, sometimes alternative therapies *do* work. Or at least, they seem to work. If you go on the website for the Healing Centre, there are lots of comments from people saying they've been helped by the healers there.'

'It could be the healers making stories up,' said Jaz, 'or only posting the positive comments they get and deleting any complaints. But even so, it's just people's biased opinions about their own experiences. It's not scientific evidence. Maybe they didn't actually have the disease they thought they had, because they didn't go to a doctor and get a proper diagnosis, so they didn't *truly* get healed by homeopathy or whatever it was. Or maybe the patients were seeing a doctor at the same time, and when they were cured, they assumed it was due to homeopathy when it was really due to the medicine the doctor prescribed.'

'And maybe the disease was going to get better anyway,' said Rosy slowly. 'Remember Hippocrates saying every disease has a crisis point? What if people only go out and get help from an alternative healer when their disease is at its worst? So, at that point, they're either going to get better or they're going to die, whatever kind of treatment they have. If they die, they obviously won't be writing any comments on websites. But if they get better, they might think the alternative therapy cured them, when really it had no effect at all.'

'That's a common mistake people make,' said Alison, coming into the room and dumping her satchel on her desk, 'even though correlation does not equal causation.'

This was the sort of incomprehensible statement her mother often made and which Rosy usually ignored, but now she was interested enough to ask what Alison meant.

'Just because two things happen together doesn't mean that one of them caused the other,' explained Alison. 'It could be a coincidence. Or it could be that they're both related to something else, which is the

Chapter Twelve

real cause. For example, let's say a study finds that the more often teenage girls wear navy pleated skirts, the more likely it is that they'll need treatment for a knee injury. So we can say that wearing navy pleated skirts has a strong *correlation* with knee injuries. But putting on a navy pleated skirt doesn't *cause* knee injuries. It's just that navy pleated skirts are often part of a netball uniform and netball is a sport that tends to cause knee injuries. If you want to find out if a treatment is truly responsible for curing a disease, you need to do a proper trial using –'

'Yeah, yeah, randomised treatment groups,' said Rosy, 'and controlling for any variables that might affect your results.'

'And analysing all your data carefully,' said Jaz, 'using wonderful, amazing, magnificent MATHS.' Then she ducked as Rosy threw a cushion at her head.

'The problem *is* that a lot of people don't really understand how science works,' said Alison.

'Well, whose fault is that?' said Rosy. 'Scientists!'

'Yes, I know,' Alison conceded. 'We could be doing a much better job at educating the public. But it's difficult. People who are brilliant at doing experiments in the lab aren't necessarily going to be brilliant at explaining their research to non-scientists. And magazines and TV shows would much rather interview a Hollywood actress going on about how blueberries cure cancer than a boring old scientist explaining why the scientific evidence for that doesn't stack up. Unfortunately, the media likes simple, quick, unchanging explanations and science doesn't work that way.'

Alison paused, then went on. 'Actually, maybe *that's* why people are attracted to things like homeopathy. A doctor would never promise that a treatment would be completely successful with no side effects, but a homeopath would. If patients are given a guarantee they'll be cured, they feel more in control and less stressed. It makes them feel better instantly – especially when the homeopath is also telling them how unique and special they are and how holistic and natural the treatment is.'

'It's more like religion than science,' said Jaz.

'Exactly. Where faith and rituals and tradition are more important than facts and evidence,' said Alison.

'Yeah, well,' said Rosy, rather grumpily, feeling outnumbered, 'it's not as though conventional medicine is perfect.'

CHAPTER THIRTEEN

*'Cured yesterday of my disease,
I died last night of my physician.'*
  ~ *Matthew Prior*

Rosy had had an excellent weekend. She and Alison had spent Saturday morning at the local markets, where they'd found two framed posters for Alison's flat and Rosy had bought a squashy rainbow-coloured ball for Reuben and some postcards to send to her friends from school, along with a tiny wooden easel that was exactly the right size to display Dr Huxley's St Vitus icon and only cost her fifty cents. Then they'd caught the bus down to Circular Quay and eaten fish and chips on the harbour steps, fending off marauding seagulls and watching the ferries churn past the great white sails of the Opera House.

'And then we walked around to the Art Gallery, which was awesome,' Rosy told Jaz. 'You could have come with us! I'd have asked you earlier if I'd known your dad was coming in to work on Saturday.'

'I couldn't anyway,' said Jaz. 'I had to visit ... I mean, I had family stuff on.'

'Oh, okay. Hang on, I need more polish.'

Jaz held out the bottle. They were nearing the end of the second-floor banisters, having worked their shiny magic all the way up the main staircase and along the floor below, where Ferdinand and his wife were currently whisking in and out of rooms with armfuls of sheets and towels. Rosy, feeling a bit guilty about the yellow pellets that were still turning up in odd corners of the college, had offered to help with the preparations for the conference visitors.

'Did you find out what this conference is about?' asked Jaz.

'Oh, yeah,' said Rosy. 'It's Big Pharma.'

'Big Farmer?' said Jaz. 'You mean, agriculture?'

'No, drugs. It's some big international pharmaceutical company having its annual meeting. "Big Pharma" – that's what my dad always calls those sort of companies.'

'Hmm. Interesting coincidence,' said Jaz. 'Because Dr Huxley's next object is the Aspro box.'

'Coincidence … or *fate*?'

'Coincidence. Hey, do we need to keep going?' Jaz gestured around the corner with her cloth.

'No, that's where they're fixing the lights. No one's staying in that wing. It can stay unpolished. Good thing, too, my arm's about to drop off with exhaustion.'

'Then let's go to your room and – Oh! What happened with your Midnight Visitor last night?'

'Phase One of my experiment went off without a hitch,' said Rosy proudly. 'Well, almost without a hitch – it was pretty hot in there with the window locked.

Chapter Thirteen

But so far, everything is proceeding according to my hypothesis. I'm initiating Phase Two tonight.'

'Can't you at least give me a *tiny* clue?'

'Nope,' said Rosy. 'I'm not releasing any results until I've analysed all my data.'

They stashed their supplies in the cleaner's cupboard, then climbed the tower stairs to Rosy's room, where they settled at her desk.

'Right, so I found out "Aspro" is just a brand name for aspirin, which has been around for ages,' said Jaz, digging in her bag for her notes. 'The story's quite exciting, actually.'

'Really?' said Rosy. 'So it involves stolen treasures, revolutionaries, secret agents and evil masterminds, does it?'

'Yes,' said Jaz. 'Also, explosions.'

Rosy raised both eyebrows. 'Oh, all right, then. Cool.' She tapped Methuselah into life. 'Carry on.'

'Well, it all began one day in 1757, when an English clergyman called Edward Stone was walking by the river near his home. He looked at the willow trees and decided to tear off a piece of bark and eat it.'

'As you do.'

'No, that bit didn't make a whole lot of sense to me, either,' admitted Jaz. 'But he was interested in finding a cure for ague, which is what they called malaria, and I guess most medicines came from plants in those days. And Paracelsus had a theory that Nature would always provide a cure close to the cause of an illness. Like, if you got stung by nettles, you could usually find some dock leaves nearby to soothe the pain. Ague seemed to be caused by marshland and willows grew near water, so maybe willows could cure ague. And when Edward Stone tasted the willow bark, it was bitter, just like a powdered bark called cinchona that was used to treat ague.'

'Hey, that's the bark that inspired Samuel Hahnemann to invent homeopathy!'

'Yes, but unlike homeopathy, cinchona actually worked. The problem was that it was really expensive because it had to be shipped all the way from Peru. So Edward dried some willow bark and tried it on people in his village who were suffering from ague and their fevers went away. What he didn't know was that willow bark contains a natural form of aspirin, which brings down high temperatures and stops aches and pains.'

Rosy interrupted again. 'Hang on, didn't the ancient Egyptians use willow in their medicine? Remember, Naomi said they put it on infected wounds.'

'They used willow *leaves*, which have hardly any active drug in them and not much of it can get absorbed through the skin, anyway. Willow also turns up in the ancient medical texts of Hippocrates and Celsus and Dioscorides and Galen, but most of what they wrote about it was rubbish. In any case, people had forgotten all that by the eighteenth century. But thanks to Edward, people in England started using willow bark for fevers and by the 1830s, some scientists had found the active ingredient in it, which they called salicylic acid.

Chapter Thirteen

'Not only that, but a Swiss apothecary called Johann Pagenstecher extracted the same substance from the meadowsweet flowers that grew near his house. The only problem was that salicylic acid caused terrible stomach problems. Fortunately, some German chemists came up with an easy way of changing its chemical structure to turn it into acetylsalicylic acid, which was even more effective as a medicine and didn't have those awful side effects. They named it "aspirin" and their company, Bayer, took out a patent so that no one else could sell it.'

'Interesting,' said Rosy, 'but so far, there's a distinct lack of criminal masterminds and explosions in your story.'

'Well, Bayer was pretty forceful about stopping anyone else in the world selling aspirin. Then the First World War broke out, with Germany fighting against Britain and its allies, which led to the Great Phenol Plot.'

'This sounds more promising.'

'Phenol was a chemical needed to make aspirin, but it's also a key ingredient of explosives. The war caused a severe phenol shortage, but Germany sent a secret agent – who'd worked at Bayer – to the United States to set up a fake company and buy lots of American phenol. Except one of the Germans accidentally left his briefcase full of incriminating documents on a train, and the US Secret Service agent who was following him picked it up. So the plot was uncovered, and the Americans got really annoyed with Bayer and ended up confiscating Bayer's aspirin factory in New York.'

'But nothing actually exploded? Not even the briefcase?'

'No, but there were quite a few explosions in Australia. You see, once the war started, Australia couldn't buy anything from German companies and a severe aspirin shortage developed. So a pharmacist in Melbourne called George Nicholas and his inventor friend, Henry Woolf Shmith, decided to make their own. They didn't have any proper scientific equipment, so they had to use pots and pans from the kitchen and … um … they had a few failures. Explosive failures. But eventually they figured out a new method of making pure aspirin crystals. They couldn't call it "aspirin" because Bayer owned that name, so they decided on "Aspro". Then they came up with lots of clever ways to mass-produce and package and market the tablets, and Aspro became a global brand.'

'Hmm,' said Rosy. 'What about criminal masterminds?'

'There was the Aspirin Ring Gang in 1927. Aspirin was so valuable in those days that a criminal gang broke into a warehouse in New York and stole a million aspirin tablets. And when the gang got caught, they kidnapped a witness's family and tried to bribe the jury.'

'That *is* quite dramatic.'

'Also, I believe you mentioned revolutionaries? How about the Russian Revolution of 1917?'

'Oh, come on. How is *that* related to aspirin?' said Rosy.

Chapter Thirteen

'The Russian Tsar's only son and heir had haemophilia, which causes uncontrollable bleeding. Doctors prescribed lots of aspirin for the pain, but what they didn't know is that aspirin stops blood clotting, so they actually made the poor boy's condition much worse. The family were so desperate that they turned to an evil monk called Rasputin, who claimed to have all sorts of healing powers. Rasputin stopped the boy taking aspirin, little Alexei felt better, Rasputin gained huge influence over the royal family, the Russians got fed up with the Tsar and killed the whole family, and the first Communist state was established, with Communism eventually spreading throughout the world.'

'Yeah, I don't think you can really blame Communism on *aspirin* …'

'Also, Bayer was part of a German corporation that helped Hitler come to power, used slave labour in its chemical factories, and manufactured the gas used to murder people in Nazi concentration camps.'

'Okay. That is truly horrible.'

'One more interesting fact about Bayer. When their chemists first came up with a way of making aspirin, the head of their department wasn't very interested in it, because there was another medicine he was working on that seemed far more useful. It was not only a highly effective painkiller and cough medicine, but it also made the people who tried it feel really good – made them feel "heroic", actually. So guess what they decided to call this drug?'

'What?'
'Heroin.'

Over lunch in Alison's flat, Rosy continued her attack on Big Pharma.

'I mean, selling heroin! As a cough mixture! Giving it to *children*!'

'Well, Bayer did take it off the market when they realised how addictive it was,' said Jaz.

'Yeah, *twelve years* after they started selling it! Oh, and while we're on the subject of medical disasters caused by pharmaceutical companies, what about thalidomide, eh?'

'That was given to pregnant women, wasn't it?' said Jaz. 'For morning sickness.'

'Yes, and then their poor babies died or were born with all sorts of deformities, like having no arms or legs! And that was in the 1960s or something. Scientists should have known better by then.'

'The problem was that Chemie Grünenthal, the German company that made thalidomide, *didn't* use science,' said Alison. 'They did the bare minimum of testing on animals before thalidomide went on the market. They didn't bother to test the drug on pregnant animals. They didn't do any controlled studies on humans. Some of their employees who'd taken the drug gave birth to children with deformities, but the company ignored that.

Chapter Thirteen

'It wasn't until a couple of years later that a doctor in Germany and another in Australia noticed the connection between thalidomide and birth defects, and even then, Grünenthal kept insisting that their drug was safe. It took fifty years for the company to offer an apology to thalidomide survivors and their families. Grünenthal seemed more interested in making money and avoiding legal responsibility than helping sick people or doing good scientific research.'

'But there are rules now, aren't there, to stop pharmaceutical companies doing that?' said Jaz.

'Yes, that was the one good thing to come out of the thalidomide tragedy, that governments around the world started taking the issue seriously,' said Alison. 'Nowadays, pharmaceutical companies have to prove their medicine is effective and safe before they're allowed to sell it. They're supposed to tell the truth when they're marketing it to doctors and pharmacists, and they need to collect data about any dangerous side effects once the public is using the medicine.

'The system's not perfect, of course, but it works most of the time. Keep in mind, though, that *all* medicines have side effects. It's just a matter of deciding how bad they are and whether the benefits outweigh any harm caused. Even thalidomide is being sold again, because it turned out to be excellent for treating leprosy and some types of cancer. As long as the patient isn't pregnant, thalidomide can be a very useful medicine.'

'Hey, and what about that Australian doctor who worked out that thalidomide caused birth defects?'

said Rosy. 'That was good work. Who was it? Someone famous now, I bet!'

'Ah, yes,' said Alison. 'William McBride.'

'What?' said Rosy, alert to the faint note of disapproval in her mother's voice. 'What did he do?'

'You know what he did,' said Alison, getting up to clear their plates. 'He noticed the link between thalidomide and birth defects in his patients. He wrote to *The Lancet* about it, won lots of awards and used his prize money to set up a medical research foundation here in Sydney.'

'And?' persisted Rosy. 'What else?'

Alison sighed. 'And he went on to do research into another medicine called Debendox, which he also thought caused birth defects. He even appeared as a witness when the manufacturer of Debendox was sued in America. Unfortunately, William McBride was later found guilty of scientific fraud.'

'Fraud?' said Jaz, wide-eyed. 'What do you mean?'

'He invented data. He'd used rabbits in one of his studies and when he wrote up the research, he increased the number of rabbits and changed the dosages so that the results said what he wanted them to say. His research assistants noticed the changes he'd made and complained about it. Eventually there were several investigations and McBride was forced to resign from his own foundation and was deregistered as a doctor.'

'He just made up stuff?' exclaimed Jaz. 'That's terrible! Why would a scientist do something like that? Especially a *famous* scientist.'

Chapter Thirteen

'He wasn't a scientist,' said Alison. 'Well, not much of one. His foundation was good at publicity, but it didn't produce much significant research. McBride was a doctor, and not all doctors are as scientific as they should be. Some of them are convinced that their own personal beliefs are far more important than scientific evidence when it comes to making decisions for their patients. I think McBride genuinely cared about preventing birth defects – remember, a number of Australian babies had been born with deformities because *he'd* given thalidomide to their mothers. You can understand why he'd want to make sure that never happened again. But inventing research results to fit your own hypothesis doesn't help.'

'It makes things *worse*,' said Rosy.

'Much worse,' Alison agreed.

'It makes people stop trusting science,' said Jaz.

CHAPTER FOURTEEN

'What is a weed? A plant whose virtues have not been discovered.'
~ *Ralph Waldo Emerson*

'It's not just aspirin that comes from Nature, you know,' said Rosy the following morning, sprawled across her bed with Methuselah as Jaz sat on the floor, sorting through the piles of library books. 'There are hundreds of plants that have been used as traditional medicines. You should see this list. Chamomile, peppermint, evening primrose, garlic, ginger, St John's wort, tea tree, valerian, cacao … Hey, that's chocolate! The Aztecs' main medicine was chocolate powder boiled with honey, vanilla and pepper. Chocolate medicine! If I were an Aztec, I'd try to get sick as often as possible.'

'Uh-huh,' said Jaz. 'Do we still need this book about the Black Death?'

Rosy glanced over. 'No. And there are lots of Australian plants used in traditional Aboriginal medicine, to heal wounds and cure stomach aches and fix sore joints. Hey, Jaz, listen, there's *scientific evidence* to support plant remedies, too. Well, some of them. For instance, it's been shown that garlic lowers blood pressure. Also, it can repel vampires.'

'What?'

'Just seeing if you were paying attention. And ginger can help with nausea, although it can also cause bleeding, and peppermint eases indigestion, except it interacts with some medicines used for heart problems.'

'Well, that makes sense,' said Jaz. 'If something's strong enough to cure an illness, it's probably strong enough to have some bad effects, too.'

'Hey, and did you know grapefruit interferes with about a *hundred* different medicines? Grapefruit! I always *knew* it was evil. Nasty, bitter stuff.'

'What, you mean taking medicine with grapefruit juice stops the medicine working?'

'No, it makes it work *too* much,' said Rosy. 'There's this chemical in grapefruit that stops your body breaking down certain medicines, so then the medicine builds up quickly in your blood and you can easily overdose on it. There was one patient who had kidney failure after eating too much marmalade.'

'Oh, here's another medicine made from plants,' said Jaz, who'd become a bit sidetracked and had started reading the books she was supposed to be organising. 'Digitalis, made from dried foxglove leaves. William Withering published *An Account of the Foxglove and Some of its Medical Uses* in 1785, after nine years of experiments. Foxglove was used for heart problems at first, but then for conditions like epilepsy, asthma and insanity as well. Even now, doctors sometimes prescribe it for congestive heart failure, although not very often, because it has some very weird side effects.

Chapter Fourteen

Apparently, if you take too much, you see halos around things and the world turns yellow –'

'Wait, what was that?' said Rosy, sitting up. 'Yellow? Halos? What plant did you say caused that?'

'Foxglove. Why?'

'Vincent!' Rosy had dived off the bed and was rooting through her bag. 'Vincent van Gogh! When you look at his paintings, you can see – Oh, here it is.' She held up a large book. 'I got this for Christmas from Dad and Gabrielle. Vincent van Gogh is my favourite painter of all time. But here, look at this. Just before he died, he painted his doctor sitting at a table with a vase of foxglove. And here's a second portrait of Dr Gachet, holding another stalk of foxglove!'

'Isn't this the artist who cut off his own ear?' Jaz frowned at the page. 'Maybe the doctor was using foxglove as a treatment for insanity.'

'Yes, and maybe the dose was a bit too strong because, look!' Rosy showed Jaz painting after painting of wheat fields, of haystacks, of sunflowers. 'All yellow!'

'But … what other colour would you paint sunflowers?' said Jaz.

Rosy gave her a pitying look. 'You can paint them any colour you like. Especially if you're Vincent van Gogh. Purple, green, blue, anything. But look. *The Yellow House*. *The Night Café*. The furniture in his bedroom. All yellow. Now look at *The Starry Night*.'

She pointed to the fuzzy golden stars swirling through the night sky and the bright yellow moon with its blurred halo.

'I've just come up with a brilliant theory about Vincent van Gogh's painting techniques,' said Rosy. 'It was the result of too much foxglove!'

'Um ... yeah,' said Jaz. 'Do you think we should be going now? We don't want to keep your mum waiting.' Alison was taking them out for lunch because the refectory was still overrun by Big Pharma representatives. Jaz's dad had been invited to lunch, too, but he said he was waiting for some trees to be delivered.

'I will probably become extremely famous now, thanks to my theory,' Rosy said, putting on her sandals. 'But don't worry, I won't forget who inspired my brainwave. I'll mention your name in a footnote.'

'Gee, thanks,' said Jaz.

They walked to Alison's office via the shop, where they bought more cream paper to print out their research.

'That's the problem with history,' said Rosy. 'There's so much of it. It just goes on and on, doesn't it?'

But Jaz was gazing across the road. 'There's the Faculty of Pharmacy. I hadn't noticed that before.'

'Let's go in and have a look,' said Rosy, dragging Jaz over the road and through the front doors of the old white building. 'Don't worry, we've got loads of time ... Ooh, check this out!' A large cabinet held a display of old medicine bottles and porcelain urns. 'They really knew how to name medicines in the olden days, didn't they? "Blue Pills". "Grey Powder". "UNG. AC. BOR." – that's really catchy. No, wait, here's a good one: "Coffee-Mint".'

Chapter Fourteen

'That sounds more like a lolly than a medicine,' said Jaz. 'What about this, "Ferrous Carbonate et Strychnine"? Strychnine! That's a really dangerous poison!'

Rosy had turned around to examine the framed prints hanging on the walls, which depicted the history of pharmacy. The first showed an elderly Chinese man sitting cross-legged on a straw mat, examining a handful of herbs. This was followed by some women from ancient Greece, rolling out medicinal clay tablets and stamping them with an official seal, and then –

'Oh no,' said Rosy. 'You can't escape him. He's everywhere.' A brawny figure in a sky-blue toga was holding out an open jar to a young woman, who was smearing white ointment on her arm. 'Hey, ladies! It is I, Galen, inventor of Miracle Beauty Cream! All who use my cream become stunningly beautiful, except those who turn purple, swell up like a balloon and explode, which they were going to do anyway!'

'Look at him!' said Jaz, starting to giggle. 'He's just so … so *smug*.'

After this, it became impossible to keep a straight face. Each picture contained something that set them off, whether it was the goofy expressions of the camels outside the eighth-century Arabic apothecary shop, or the pigeons lurking gleefully behind the medieval monks tending a medicinal herb garden, or the awkward, splay-legged pose of the Renaissance scribe helping to compile an official reference book of medicines.

By the final picture, 'Pharmacy Today and Tomorrow', they'd lost it completely. A square-jawed young man in a crisp white lab coat stared solemnly into the future, while an older man patted him on the shoulder. Pharmacy, the label informed them, would continue, its traditions passed down 'from father to son'. The supposedly futuristic equipment – a stainless-steel scale and some orange glassware – appeared to be from the 1960s.

'They need some flying saucers in the background,' gasped Rosy. 'Everyone should be wearing jetpacks. There should be a robot in a frilly apron to dust their benchtop.'

'Stop it,' begged Jaz. 'Someone will hear us. Oh, my ribs. Come on, let's go.'

They staggered outside and by the time they reached Alison's office, they were reasonably composed, although a glimpse through a doorway of Marcus in a lab coat ('He looks like the Future of Pharmacy,' whispered Rosy) resulted in a lot of undignified snorting. Alison gave them a quelling look, then led them out the doors, across the park and down some narrow streets to a tiny Vietnamese restaurant.

Here they sat at a counter in the window and chased slippery noodles around bowls of steaming broth with their chopsticks. Across the road was a shopfront with a sign advertising Traditional Chinese Medicine, which prompted Rosy to tell Alison about the legendary Shen Nung, who'd tested hundreds of plants on himself to discover their medicinal powers and had thus become the founder of Chinese Pharmacy. Alison did not seem very impressed.

Chapter Fourteen

'Well, Chinese people have been using those remedies for thousands of years, so they must have *some* effect,' said Rosy.

'Just because something's traditional, doesn't mean it works,' said Alison.

'Yes, look at bloodletting,' said Jaz, because she always agreed with Alison.

'Just because it's old, doesn't mean it *doesn't* work,' Rosy retorted. 'I mean, has anyone done any scientific testing on it?'

'Yes,' said Alison. 'Quite a few studies have been done on both Chinese herbal remedies and acupuncture, as well as other traditional therapies. Unfortunately, there's very little evidence that any of them are effective. And overall, the quality of the research is very poor. There are hardly any large, randomised, double-blind, placebo-controlled trials.'

'What's double-blind?'

'Where neither the patient nor the doctor know whether someone's getting the medicine or a placebo. Double-blinding means there's less chance that the doctor or the patient will be biased when reporting their results.'

'Oh, right,' said Rosy. 'Although you couldn't really do placebo acupuncture, anyway.'

'Yes, you can,' said Alison. 'You can use fake needles that only scratch the skin or you can stick the needles in places that acupuncture theory says won't have any effect. Acupuncture was found to help with some types of pain, but when researchers compared actual acupuncture to placebo acupuncture, they found there was very little difference. Plus, acupuncture isn't always harmless. Dirty needles can cause infections, a needle pushed too far in the wrong place can puncture a lung –'

'But regular doctors can do that, too,' said Rosy. 'Patients are always getting infections in hospitals or having medical instruments accidentally sewn up inside them during operations.'

'True, and mistakes can be made when prescribing conventional medicines,' said Alison. 'But at least there are rules in place to try to prevent these problems. Traditional treatments are far less regulated and precise. If traditional healers use a dried plant, they have no idea how much active ingredient is in that particular set of leaves, so it's easy to get the dosage wrong. One Chinese remedy was found to have killed dozens of people from heart attacks and strokes, and another caused kidney failure. And some of them have been found to be contaminated with lead, mercury, arsenic – all sorts of toxic substances.'

Alison was in full-blown lecturer mode by now and a few of the surrounding diners stopped slurping noodles to listen in.

'In addition,' Alison continued, waving her chopstick around, 'many traditional Chinese remedies use animal ingredients that are not only ineffective, but threaten the existence of endangered species. Rhinos are on their way to extinction now because their horns are in demand for useless Chinese remedies. Then

Chapter Fourteen

there are horribly cruel practices like draining live bears of their bile –'

'Big Pharma does horrible animal testing, too,' said Rosy. 'They're *both* wrong. And I can't believe that, out of all those hundreds of Chinese herbal medicines, none of them do anything useful.'

'Artemisinin,' said a bespectacled man beside them. 'Extracted from sweet wormwood, a traditional remedy for malaria. Chinese researchers tested it in the 1960s and found it was more effective than any other known malaria medicine. Now it's part of the standard treatment for malaria.'

'Thanks! There you go,' said Rosy, turning to Alison. 'See? Medicine manufactured by Nature.'

'And then improved by Science,' said Jaz, who always had to have the last word.

CHAPTER FIFTEEN

'In science, the credit goes to the man who convinces the world, not to the man to whom the idea first occurs.'
  ~ *Francis Darwin*

Rosy and Jaz arrived back at New College to find a small crowd gathered on the front steps, watching a half-grown eucalypt being manoeuvred into a hole.

'The garden's looking good, isn't it?' said Lynette to Mohammad the security guard, as Jaz's dad began shovelling dirt around the bundle of tree roots. 'It'll be lovely when it's finished. We just need a bit of rain.'

They all automatically tipped their heads back to scan the bare blue skies.

'There's a sort of wispy cloud over there, I think,' said Rosy, gazing into the distance.

'That's smoke from the hospital incinerator,' snapped Ms Boydell. Maybe she was worried about the cost of watering all these new plants. She certainly didn't look like someone wanting to spend any more money on the college gardens.

'Well, they say there'll be a break in the weather by the end of the week ...' said Lynette doubtfully, then she brightened. 'Oh, that reminds me! The lawyer looking after Dr Huxley's bequest rang. He's coming out on Friday afternoon.'

Rosy and Jaz shot each other looks of alarm.

'I'm sure he'll be thrilled when he sees all the labels you girls have made,' Lynette went on cheerfully. 'Just let me know if you need to use our laminating machine –'

But Rosy and Jaz were gone, racing off through the foyer and up the stairs to the Senior Common Room.

'Don't panic, we've only got four more objects to go,' said Rosy to Jaz, who was peering anxiously into the cabinet. 'Three, if we chuck out that mouldy old medallion.'

'We are *not* throwing out any of Dr Huxley's collection,' said Jaz. 'Do you have the key?'

Rosy handed it over and Jaz unlocked the cabinet and drew out the next object – the framed medallion in its leather case.

'That's definitely paper underneath the glass,' said Rosy. 'Paper covered in *mould*. See, it's all green and fuzzy.' Then she looked at it again. 'Hey, Jaz? Last week, did you actually take this thing out of its case and turn it over to see the back?'

'Well, no, because – Rosy! What are you doing? Don't! You'll break it!'

'It's not that fragile. And look, I can run my fingernail all the way around, between it and the case. It's not *totally* wedged in there …'

'No, I really don't think you should!'

Rosy gave her a stern look. 'What kind of scientist are you, if you're not prepared to take a risk to discover something new? Do you think William Harvey would have hesitated? Or Louis Pasteur? I mean, come on – what would Emily Rosa do?'

'Okay, okay!' said Jaz. 'Just … be careful …'

They both held their breath as Rosy carefully prised the medallion out and turned it over.

'Aha!' said Rosy. 'Writing!'

Unfortunately, it was old-fashioned handwriting in very faded brown ink. They bent their heads over it, trying to decipher the words.

'Is that a "u"? No, that would make it "nuued",' said Jaz.

'Or "muuld".'

'I'm sure that third line says "which makes".'

'And the date is "1948". But what's that long loopy word on the fourth line?'

Jaz suddenly clapped her hands. 'I've got it! Penicillin! "The mould which makes Penicillin"!'

'Penicillin?' said Rosy. 'Isn't that an antibiotic? Hey, and antibiotics were a very important development in medicine! I bet that's why Dr Huxley wanted this in his collection.'

'Yes, and penicillin is made from *mould*! Mouldy bread or something like that!'

'There you go,' said Rosy, sitting back. 'Didn't I *say* that it was mould?'

'Didn't you say we should chuck the whole thing out?' countered Jaz. 'What's that signature above the date?'

'A … lemming,' said Rosy. 'Okay, probably not. But whoever it was, I wish they'd learned how to write neatly.'

'Let's go and look it up,' said Jaz, and after securing the medallion in the cabinet, they ran upstairs to Rosy's room.

'Alexander Fleming,' announced Jaz presently, head buried in one of her books. 'In 1928, he discovered mould on one of his Petri dishes and noticed it was dissolving the bacteria he'd been trying to grow.'

Meanwhile, Rosy had been busy with Methuselah. 'Ahem!' she said. 'And note that he only discovered this because he left his workbench cluttered with old Petri dishes for weeks at a time. The benefits of a messy room demonstrated, *yet again*.'

'Yeah, well, his lab might have been a bit untidy, but he was very observant and *organised*,' said Jaz. 'He identified the mould and spent years growing it and testing it to show that it really did kill certain bacteria, without harming animals. And, of course, chance favours only the *prepared* mind. He'd never have paid any attention to that mould's actions if he hadn't already discovered that lysosomes found in humans can kill bacteria.'

'Urgh.' Rosy pulled a face. 'And have you read *how* he discovered lysosomes? He had a cold and he experimented with some of his own snot in a Petri dish! And when he realised his snot could kill bacteria, he went around asking his workmates for snot samples so he could test those as well!'

'That is a perfectly valid form of scientific enquiry,' said Jaz, trying not to look disgusted.

Rosy started laughing. 'And then he found *tears* were the best source of lysosomes! And when his colleagues ran out of patience with his demands for their tears, he paid small boys to cry for him! Oh, oh, listen – he actually tried to collect tears from farm animals! But the pigs refused to cooperate!'

'Can we please get back to penicillin?' said Jaz. 'Are you taking notes?'

'No, I'm laughing too much. I'm *crying* with laughter. Bacteria are dying all over the place.'

'Stop it. Now, write this down. Fleming managed to produce some mould juice, which was an unstable and impure form of penicillin, and a colleague of his, Cecil Paine, found that mould juice cleared up eye infections. But Paine didn't publish his results and Fleming didn't know enough about chemistry to be able to make any pure, stable penicillin. Fleming gave up. What he really needed was –'

'An Australian!' said Rosy. 'Howard Florey!'

'What he needed was a *team*. Not just Howard Florey, who was a pathologist and pharmacologist, but Ernst Chain, a German biochemist, and Norman Heatley, a British biochemist, and lots of other scientists working together at Oxford, including Margaret Jennings and Jean Orr-Ewing. They were the first to isolate pure penicillin from mould after reading about Fleming's discovery. *They* were the ones who first tested this new medicine on a human and proved it worked. They gave it to a man who was dying of a terrible infection after he'd been … been …'

'Scratched by a thorn while gardening!' cried Rosy. They jumped up and leaned out the window over the front garden, where Jaz's dad was now spreading manure with a dangerously sharp-looking shovel. Jaz opened her mouth to shout a warning, but Rosy grabbed her. 'No, don't, you might startle him,' she said. 'Anyway, it's okay – penicillin's been invented now. That cures infections.'

Jaz allowed Rosy to tug her away from the window, although she still looked worried. 'But that other gardener *died*,' she said.

'Only because they didn't have enough penicillin at that stage to treat him for more than a few days,' said Rosy consolingly. 'It worked really well as long as their supplies held out.'

Actually, Florey's team had been reduced to collecting the poor patient's urine, separating out the penicillin and then reusing it on him, but Rosy didn't think it would be helpful to point this out. She decided to distract Jaz with some other, less revolting, facts.

'Then they took penicillin to America,' she said, 'and American scientists worked out how to mass-produce it – which was handy, because it was the Second World War and they needed lots of penicillin to treat wounded soldiers. And then Fleming, Florey and Chain were awarded the Nobel Prize.' Rosy frowned. 'Actually, that's not very fair. What about Norman Heatley and Margaret Jennings and the rest of them at Oxford? What about those Americans, Andrew Moyer and his team? How come they missed out on the prize?'

'It's against the rules for more than three people to share a Nobel Prize,' said Jaz, her attention successfully diverted back to her book. 'Anyway, Fleming wasn't even the first to realise that mould could kill bacteria.

Chapter Fifteen

It says here that Joseph Lister, Louis Pasteur and lots of other scientists – including Thomas Huxley – had already noticed that. Even the ancient Greeks used mouldy bread on infected wounds. But the good thing was that scientists started looking for other types of natural antibiotics. Schatz and Waksman discovered streptomycin in soil and Brotzu discovered cephalosporin in, um … raw sewage.'

'That's true dedication to medical science,' said Rosy. 'Spending years searching through sewage.'

'Oh, and Domagk discovered that chemicals called sulfonamides could treat infections, too. But I guess that's not really a natural antibiotic because they came from artificial dyes –'

'Hey, it's Marcus!' interrupted Rosy, staring out the window. 'What's he doing here?'

'Maybe he's looking for your mum,' said Jaz. At the moment, though, Marcus appeared to be deep in conversation with Jaz's dad, who was leaning on his shovel and pointing at some of the new native flowers he'd planted. Rosy and Jaz raised their eyebrows at each other, then hurried downstairs to investigate.

'Ah, there they are,' said Marcus, catching sight of them. 'Well, I'll let you get back to your work,' he said to Jaz's dad. 'Good to chat with you.'

'What were you talking about?' asked Jaz, at the same time Rosy said, 'Chat about what?'

'None of your beeswax, Scooby Gang,' said Marcus. 'Here, can you give this to Dr Radford?'

'She's gone into the city,' said Rosy, accepting the folder he held out.

'Yeah, I know that, Scooby-Doo. She's at a committee meeting. She asked if I'd pick this up from the lab and drop it in here on my way home. Although it's probably *safer* to leave it with the ladies in the office –'

'I am very trustworthy!' said Rosy, hugging the folder tighter. 'I'll put it on her desk. And I'm not Scooby-Doo. I'm the cool one, I'm Daphne.'

Meanwhile, Jaz had been studying Marcus's T-shirt, which today depicted a couple of snarling yellow blobs. A speech bubble from an adjacent orange blob contained the words, 'Resistance is futile!'

'I don't get it,' said Jaz.

'What? Oh,' said Marcus, glancing down at his shirt. 'The yellow ones are meant to be MRSA. Methicillin-resistant *Staphylococcus aureus*. You know, superbugs?' He turned to Rosy. '*You* know about antibiotic resistance, right? I mean, given your mother is a world-renowned expert in the subject? And has just been appointed chief scientific adviser to a federal government body set up to deal with the problem?'

'Um ...' said Rosy, feeling both ignorant and guilty. Maybe she should have been paying a bit more attention whenever Alison discussed her work. But of course, *Jaz* knew what he was on about.

'Alexander Fleming talked about penicillin resistance in his Nobel Prize speech,' Jaz said. 'Is that the same thing?'

'That's it,' said Marcus. 'Within a couple of years of penicillin being released, it'd stopped killing some bacteria. Scientists discovered new antibiotics, but the same thing happened again, with an even wider

Chapter Fifteen

range of bacteria. Now there are superbugs that can't be killed by *any* known antibiotic. Too bad if you get infected with one of those bugs the next time you go into hospital.'

'But why?' said Rosy. 'Why did the antibiotics stop working?'

'Okay. Imagine there are a whole lot of one type of bacteria,' said Marcus. 'Say, *Staph. aureus*, the round yellow ones, and they're hanging about inside someone, causing an infection. Hit them with a huge dose of penicillin and they'll all die. But let's say you don't use *enough* penicillin. Maybe the patient with the infection only takes half the packet of tablets, then stops, because he feels better. Now, nearly all of the *Staph. aureus* have died, but there are just a few that happen to be strong enough to survive that low dose of penicillin. Those are the bacteria that are left to reproduce. They pass on their strong penicillin-resistant genes to the next generation of bacteria. Eventually, those bacteria are the only ones around and penicillin doesn't do a thing to them.'

'Is that how antibiotic resistance starts?' said Jaz. 'People not taking all of their medication?'

'Well, it certainly doesn't help, but no, that's not the main cause of the problem,' said Marcus. 'It was always going to happen, but it's made much worse by overusing antibiotics. Doctors often prescribe them for patients who have viral infections like a cold or the flu, even though antibiotics are useless against viruses. Patients demand antibiotics for all sorts of ridiculous things and they get them. In parts of Asia and Africa, you can buy antibiotics in shops without a prescription, in doses so small that they're guaranteed to do nothing but cause antibiotic resistance – which is why places like India and Thailand have such huge numbers of superbugs. Then travellers spread those superbugs all over the world.

'Farmers give unnecessary antibiotics to their animals, too, trying to make sure their cattle and pigs and poultry stay free of infections and grow really big. A few years back, hundreds of Americans got sick from eating hamburgers that were full of toxic *E. coli*, which used to be harmless to humans. It's not such a problem on Australian farms, but we import a lot of seafood and that's full of antibiotics and probably more than a few superbugs.'

'This is *terrible*,' said Jaz, shaking her head. 'Isn't it, Rosy?'

Rosy nodded, lips pursed, trying to look as though she'd already known about this.

'We're on the verge of a global catastrophe,' said Marcus. 'If we run out of effective antibiotics, we're back to the bad old days when people used to die of minor infections. But governments *are* starting to take the problem more seriously. There's this committee that Dr Radford's advising, for one thing. Oh, and they're funding my utterly brilliant research for another couple of years.'

'What *is* your research about?' said Jaz. 'Are you really studying honey?'

'Yep. I'm trying to find out how certain chemicals in honey kill superbugs.'

Chapter Fifteen

'Honey is an antibiotic?' said Rosy. 'So if you eat lots of honey, you're less likely to get sick?'

'Well, firstly, it's only certain types of honey. I'm studying manuka honey, made from the pollen of tea tree flowers found in Australia and New Zealand –'

'Like these?' said Jaz, pointing at a nearby bush. 'That's what you were talking to Dad about!'

'Uh-huh. And secondly, you don't *eat* it, you soak bandages in it or use it as an ointment on wounds.'

'Still, that's pretty cool, isn't it?' said Rosy. 'Another medicine provided by Nature.'

'Oh, there are lots of natural substances being tested right now,' said Marcus. 'Walnut leaves, hyacinth bulbs, camellia leaves. There's a group of Australian desert shrubs called Eremophila that have been used by Aboriginal people for thousands of years to treat infections and now we know the leaves contain chemicals that can kill MRSA. And a friend of mine in Melbourne is studying Australian tree frogs, because their skin secretions seem to be toxic to superbugs.'

'First raw sewage, now toxic frog slime?' said Rosy, with a shudder. 'Ugh. Stick with honey, Marcus.'

CHAPTER SIXTEEN

'It is those who know little, not those who know much, who so positively assert that this or that problem will never be solved by science.'
~ *Charles Darwin*

'So, what are you girls investigating this morning?' asked Alison, sticking her head round the door of Rosy's room the next day. Jaz had already spread several pages of notes over the bed and Rosy was wrestling with Methuselah's power cord, which was tangled up in the chair legs.

'Smallpox,' said Jaz.

'Vaccination,' said Rosy, from under the desk.

Alison raised her eyebrows at this, but 'Hmm' was all she said.

'What does "Hmm" mean?' asked Jaz, after Alison had gone.

'It means, "I hope you'll conduct a thorough investigation into the scientific facts about vaccination and then write a report that demolishes the so-called arguments of anti-vaccinationists",' said Rosy.

'That's a lot of information being conveyed by something that's not even a proper word.'

'My family are very skilled communicators,' said Rosy. She climbed out from underneath the desk and gazed with satisfaction at Methuselah's screen. 'There! Come and look at this, Jaz. Last night, I found photos of a smallpox vaccine packet that looks exactly like ours. It's from a science museum in London. See, "Dried Smallpox Vaccine, England, 1979". Now we don't have to open up our packet to see what's inside.'

'Good thing, too, because that stuff is highly contagious,' said Jaz. 'It's a live virus. Imagine if we accidentally dropped the glass vial and broke it.'

'It's not actually *smallpox* in the vaccine, though,' said Rosy. 'It's just cowpox, which is pretty harmless. Everyone knows that, about Edward Jenner realising that dairy maids who'd had cowpox didn't catch smallpox and then him making cowpox into a vaccine in, um ... whenever it was.'

'He published the results of his experiments in 1798,' said Jaz, consulting her notes, 'but he wasn't the first to realise that. At least six other doctors had tested cowpox vaccines already. He was just the one who did the most to publicise it. But did you know the word "vaccine" comes from the Latin word *vacca*, meaning "cow"? And that before cowpox vaccinations became common, people used to have smallpox parties where they inoculated each other with powdered smallpox scabs, taken from someone who'd had a mild form of smallpox?'

'They really knew how to have fun in the olden days, didn't they? Smallpox parties!'

Chapter Sixteen

'Obviously, it wasn't very safe,' said Jaz, 'because things could go wrong and people would end up with a fatal case of smallpox caused by the inoculation. Even the cowpox vaccine had problems. Edward Jenner sent his vaccine to a little town in Massachusetts and sixty-eight people died from it, probably because the vaccine contained the smallpox virus instead of cowpox. Then there was a German shipyard where a couple of hundred men caught hepatitis from contaminated vaccines during a smallpox vaccination campaign. But smallpox was such a horrific, deadly disease that most people felt any vaccination risks were worth it.'

'What I *still* want to know,' said Rosy, 'is why it says "NOT FOR INJECTION" on the packet.'

'Oh, that's because it's too dangerous to inject. See how there are little pronged needles included with the vial of vaccine? You dip a needle into the solution of vaccine and then scratch the person's skin with it and a blister grows on that spot. That shows the person's immune system is fighting off the virus. By the time the scab falls off, the person is protected from smallpox and cowpox. They don't use cowpox virus anymore, by the way. They use a related virus called vaccinia. It can still cause serious illness and spread to other people nearby, so hardly anyone gets this vaccine these days – not now that smallpox has been wiped out.'

'Really? There's no smallpox now, anywhere in the world?'

'There's a sample of the virus in the US and another in Russia, both locked up in high-security facilities, just in case scientists ever need to study smallpox again. But in 1980, the World Health Organization announced that the disease of smallpox had been eradicated, after a fourteen-year international vaccination campaign. It was the first time an infectious disease that killed people had been wiped out by medical science. Unfortunately, that's the *only* time, so far.'

'What about polio?' said Rosy. 'That's been eradicated, hasn't it? Or nearly. We had someone from a polio charity come to our school and talk about it.'

They looked it up on Methuselah.

'What a terrible disease,' said Jaz, staring at the screen. 'Even if you don't die or end up with withered, paralysed legs, you can still get post-polio syndrome, decades later. And look at all these epidemics in the past century, all over the world. Even in rich countries like the United States – thousands of Americans died in that 1952 epidemic.'

'Well, it was a good thing Jonas Salk invented the polio vaccine that year, wasn't it?' said Rosy. 'And then hundreds of thousands of American schoolkids were vaccinated as soon as it was released in 1955 and – Oh no.'

'One of the companies that made the vaccine hadn't killed the virus properly,' said Jaz, frowning.

'That mistake caused *forty thousand* cases of polio!' said Rosy. 'You see, *this* is why some people don't trust vaccines.'

'But that was more than sixty years ago,' said Jaz. 'They learned from that. See, it says they set up

Chapter Sixteen

regulations that mean vaccines are now safer than any other type of medicine. And then Albert Sabin developed a new vaccine that provided longer-lasting immunity.'

'And it was a drop of liquid on a sugar cube,' Rosy said. 'Much nicer than having a needle stuck in your arm. Except ... it says here it was a *live* virus.'

'Live, but not dangerous. Although then they discovered that sometimes that virus could mutate inside people and cause paralytic polio ... So they don't use that vaccine in Australia anymore – they use the one with the killed virus.'

'Good,' said Rosy, scrolling down. 'Anyway, here's the bit about polio eradication. In 1988, the World Health Organization announced they were going to wipe out polio by the year 2000. Okay, that sounds achievable – I mean, they got rid of smallpox in only fourteen years. And polio has a cheap, effective vaccine. And the virus only affects people, so they didn't have to worry about it lurking about in animals, ready to reinfect everyone. So the world went from hundreds of thousands of cases before the campaign to less than five hundred cases in 2001. But then ... what happened? Look, there were nearly two thousand cases reported in 2002.'

'That was in India,' noted Jaz, 'although then the government made a massive effort and now India is officially free of polio.'

'Good work, India! I wonder when polio ended in Australia? Let's see ... the last case was in 1972.

Excellent, that was decades ago. No, wait, then some guy arrived from Pakistan in 2007, carrying the virus!'

'I guess it doesn't matter whether individual countries are free of polio,' said Jaz, 'not while there are other countries where it's widespread. Viruses can cross borders. Polio's still around in Nigeria, Pakistan and Afghanistan, and look, all of those countries have local leaders who reckon polio vaccinations are part of an American plot to attack Muslims.'

'Hey, and remember when the Americans tracked down Osama bin Laden and killed him?' said Rosy. 'A doctor in Pakistan pretended to be giving vaccinations to the bin Laden family, when he was really spying on them for the CIA. Which probably didn't help the polio campaign.'

'Yes, but Muslim leaders in Nigeria had been boycotting vaccinations for years before that. And now the Taliban is murdering polio vaccinators in Pakistan. Oh, and there's a war in Syria, so vaccination has stopped and polio's spreading there, too. This is depressing.'

Rosy sighed. 'And it's not just the Taliban campaigning against vaccination. There are plenty of people *here* who think vaccines are evil.'

Jaz gave her a sympathetic look. 'Did your mum have an argument about vaccination with Cheryl the Homeopath?'

'No, Mum had one with Gabrielle,' said Rosy. 'And they never *usually* argue. But Gabrielle said she wasn't sure whether Reuben should have the measles vaccine and Mum called her an idiot. And Gabrielle's *not* an

Chapter Sixteen

idiot. She's really smart! She was just worried because her mothers' group watched this DVD about whether vaccines cause autism. And then she went online and found this doctor in London who'd published a scientific paper saying the measles vaccine *did* cause autism, because it isn't just the measles virus in that vaccine, it has mumps and rubella viruses in it as well, and that's all too much for babies to cope with.'

Jaz was already tapping away at Methuselah. 'Was this Dr Andrew Wakefield? Whose paper, published in *The Lancet* in 1998, linked the Measles Mumps Rubella vaccine to both bowel disease and autism?'

'Yeah, that sounds right. Although I didn't actually listen to most of their argument. Dad and I escaped to the studio and did some painting.'

'Would you like to hear about the flaws in Wakefield's research paper?'

'You're going to tell me anyway, aren't you?' said Rosy. 'Go on, then.'

'Well, firstly, his study only had twelve children in it. It wasn't even research, really. There was no control group, not even a proper hypothesis. It was just a description of some children with bowel problems and behaviour disorders, who also happened to have had the MMR vaccine, because most children *do* have the vaccine. Those twelve children weren't randomly selected from the population, either. Most of them were at his clinic because their parents wanted to find a link between autism and the MMR vaccine so they could sue someone, and the lawyers who were preparing the lawsuit against MMR were paying Wakefield.

'Also, he'd just developed his own measles vaccine that he wanted to sell, so he had a motive to attack the MMR vaccine. Then an investigation found that he'd made up data, *The Lancet* retracted his paper, and he had his medical licence taken away due to his unethical behaviour, which included doing dangerous medical tests on the children.'

'Okay, okay,' said Rosy, raising her hands in surrender.

'Meanwhile,' Jaz went on relentlessly, 'due to all this anti-MMR publicity, parents stopped vaccinating their children so there were measles outbreaks all over the place, including one in Ireland where three people died. Oh, and there have also been a number of large, well-designed studies, including one that examined data for half a million Danish children, showing no link between the MMR vaccine and autism. Are you taking notes on this?'

'No, I thought *you* were –'

There was a knock on the door and Alison walked in. Rosy groaned.

'Mum! We've got it all under control here. We don't need any of your facts!'

'What do you mean?' Alison said innocently. 'I'm simply here to ask if you want to try some of these delicious home-baked chocolate-chip cookies.'

'Yes, please!' said Jaz, jumping up, but Rosy eyed the plate warily.

'Did you make them?' she asked her mother.

'What do you think?' said Alison. 'No, of course not. Lynette did.'

Chapter Sixteen

'Oh, all right, then,' said Rosy, and she took one and it *was* delicious. Meanwhile, Alison was unabashedly craning her neck towards their notes.

'Have you got up to the thiomersal scare yet?' she asked. 'Because it's important to note that, despite the claims of certain Hollywood actresses and talk-show hosts, no children's vaccine contains any form of dangerous mercury. There's also no evidence whatsoever that vaccines cause autism, multiple sclerosis, diabetes, asthma –'

'*Mum*,' protested Rosy, but through a mouthful of molten chocolate, so it wasn't very distinct.

'Actually, I have a question,' said Jaz. 'Babies *do* get a lot of vaccinations now. Can it overload their immune systems?'

'No,' said Alison. 'Babies make a habit of eating and inhaling disgusting things – at least, Rosy did when she was a baby – but their immune systems are designed to deal with those threats very efficiently. That's the whole purpose of vaccination – it gives babies a tiny dose of an inactive virus so that if they ever get infected with the real thing, their immune system will recognise it and know how to fight it off. It's true that there are some babies with impaired immune systems – babies with AIDS or leukaemia – or with severe allergies to some of the components of vaccines. So there's always going to be a tiny number of children who can't have certain vaccines, which is why it's important that everyone *else* is immunised.'

'Is that what they mean when they talk about herd immunity?' said Jaz, looking at her notes.

Alison nodded. 'Even the best vaccine doesn't work one hundred per cent of the time. Some children who've been vaccinated will still get sick if they're exposed to that virus, although they'll probably get a much milder form of the disease than the unvaccinated children. The problem is that if fewer than ninety-five per cent of people in a community are vaccinated, the disease can still circulate. And the people most at risk of getting sick and dying are those who can't have the vaccine due to their impaired immune systems – oh, and newborns, because babies can't have most vaccines until they're at least two months old. Tiny babies are dying of whooping cough in parts of Australia where the vaccination rate has fallen below eighty per cent. That shouldn't be happening. It's due to parents ignoring scientific evidence in favour of their "mummy instinct" and it makes me very, very cross.'

'Well, you still shouldn't have called Gabrielle an idiot,' said Rosy, frowning at her mother.

'I didn't call her an idiot,' said Alison. 'I said that her *opinion* was idiotic.'

This was the sort of distinction that no doubt seemed perfectly reasonable to Alison, but made other people want to throw things at her head. Sometimes Rosy wondered not why her parents had gotten divorced, but how they'd managed to stay together as long as they had.

'Mum, you are missing the point,' said Rosy, with what she felt was a saintly amount of patience. 'Which *is* that using the word "idiot" will not make people

Chapter Sixteen

want to listen to you. Gabrielle was really upset right then. She'd just watched a program about a little boy who'd been diagnosed with autism after he had that measles vaccine and –'

'And when do most children with autism start showing signs of autistic behaviour?' said Alison. 'Oh, right, when they're between eighteen months and two years old, which just happens to be after most children have the MMR vaccine.'

'Correlation, not causation,' murmured Jaz. She was almost as bad as Alison, thought Rosy. But Alison was still going.

'You know what this reminds me of? A doctor I know told me how one day he was getting ready to inject a vaccine into a baby's arm when the baby suddenly had a seizure, right there in her mother's lap. Now, if he'd given that injection sixty seconds earlier, the mother would have been *convinced* that the vaccine was responsible for her child's epilepsy.'

Rosy gave up and ate another biscuit. (Chocolate was medicinal, right?)

'The problem *is* that all those TV programs and magazine articles about vaccination are produced by journalists who don't understand basic science,' Alison went on. 'They ignore the facts because they want to tell an enthralling story about some brave parents taking on the evil medical profession – when most doctors go into the profession to *heal* people, not to make them sick! On the rare occasion there seems to be a problem with a vaccine – as there was a few years ago here, with a flu vaccine – it gets picked up by doctors immediately and it's withdrawn from the market while more tests are done.'

Jaz was nodding vigorously as she wrote all this down. Rosy only sighed and waited for her mother to finish. She'd heard all this before.

'In a way, the story of medicine has been *too* successful,' Alison concluded. 'Parents now haven't experienced a time when children ended up in iron lungs because they'd caught polio, or were born deaf and blind because their mothers had had rubella, or when babies routinely died of measles or diphtheria or smallpox. People don't realise how *privileged* we are to have vaccines.'

'Did your brother end up having the MMR vaccine?' Jaz asked Rosy, after Alison had finally departed.

'Yes,' said Rosy. 'And no, he did not develop autism, epilepsy or asthma afterwards. He *did* steal my best coloured pencils and scribbled all over the kitchen walls and then he poured a carton of milk into the flowerbed and made mud pies and tried to eat one. But I don't think that had anything to do with the vaccine.'

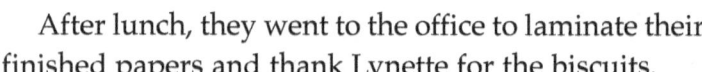

After lunch, they went to the office to laminate their finished papers and thank Lynette for the biscuits.

'They were *superb*,' said Rosy. 'They were the best chocolate-chip cookies I've ever tasted.'

'That new recipe turned out quite well, didn't it?' said Lynette, pleased. 'Maybe I should bring some in

Chapter Sixteen

on Friday afternoon, when that lawyer comes to look at your display. Dr Adam will be back from holiday then – he's the Master of the College, you know, and he's very keen to see all those things Dr Huxley bequeathed to us. We could set up the coffee machine in the common room, have a little celebration.'

'Yes!' said Rosy. 'A party!' She chose not to think about the fact that it wouldn't be much of a celebration unless she and Jaz figured out what the last two objects were. 'Chocolate-chip cookies would be *very* appropriate,' Rosy told Lynette, 'because Dr Huxley's collection is all about the history of medicine and the Aztecs believed that chocolate was medicinal.'

'Well, that makes sense,' said Lynette. 'Nothing like a cup of tea and a chocolate biscuit when you're feeling poorly.'

'Hey, and we could have salt-and-vinegar chips, too!' said Rosy. She was very fond of salt-and-vinegar chips.

'How are *they* medicinal?' said Jaz, looking up from inserting pages into plastic laminating sleeves.

'Remember, James Lind's first medical treatment trial?' said Rosy. 'He gave his scurvy patients salt water and vinegar. We could have lime cordial as well. I'll organise the chips and cordial, Lynette.'

'I must invite Dr Bennet, too,' said Lynette. 'I'll give her a ring this afternoon.'

'And can we ask a couple of people who've helped us?' said Rosy. 'Naomi at the Nicholson Museum? She's an expert in ancient Egyptian medicine. And also the flying fox lady from the Macleay Museum?'

'And your mum,' said Jaz. 'And Marcus.'

'Marcus! Yeah, all right then, he can come. And we have to invite your dad, too, Jaz. And what about your –' She checked herself, as she'd nearly mentioned Jaz's mysteriously missing mum. 'Your cousins and your auntie and uncle?' Rosy finished hurriedly.

'Rajindar and Tej will be at work, Kirin's at tennis camp –'

'Just give me a list by Friday morning,' said Lynette, 'so I know how many coffee cups to put out.'

'Rosy, come and give me a hand with this machine,' ordered Jaz, so Rosy had to abandon her party plans for the moment. But the laminating machine, like most of the equipment in the office, was as old and sluggish as Methuselah, and they had quite a few pages to do. As Rosy stood there, watching the machine plod along, her thoughts turned to her Midnight Visitor. She'd planned to initiate Phase Three of her experiment that night, but she still had a few technical difficulties to overcome. It was tempting to discuss the problem with Jaz – after all, it was teamwork, not individual brilliance, that had led to that breakthrough with penicillin – but Rosy desperately wanted to solve this mystery by herself. She was suddenly struck by an idea.

'Do you have a list of which students stayed in which rooms last year?' she asked Lynette. 'I mean, do you know who was in my room?'

'Did they leave something in there?' said Lynette. 'Bring it down and I'll put it in the Lost Property box.'

'No, I just wondered ... I mean, I don't need to know their name or anything, but could you look up what they were studying?'

Chapter Sixteen

'You're in the front tower room, aren't you?' Lynette pulled out one of her folders. 'Oh, yes, I remember. It was that nice girl from the country, the one doing Vet Science.'

'Aha!' said Rosy.

The evidence was piling up in favour of her hypothesis. All she needed now was incontrovertible proof. If *only* Methuselah could be trusted to run his camera all night! But he was bound to overheat and switch himself off and probably set the desk on fire while he was at it ... Rosy sighed, her gaze wandering idly about the office. It landed on Lynette's desk, which held a plate, empty now except for a sprinkling of cookie crumbs. Rosy's eyes widened.

'All done,' said Jaz, gathering up their laminated papers. 'Want to put these up in the common room now?'

'Sure,' said Rosy. 'I just need to grab a couple of things from the kitchen first, though.' An apple, for one. And some flour.

CHAPTER SEVENTEEN

'Mystics exult in mystery and want it to stay mysterious. Scientists exult in mystery for a different reason: it gives them something to do.'
~ Richard Dawkins

'Guess what?' Rosy and Jaz shouted at each other, as Jaz burst through Rosy's doorway the following morning.

'What?' said Rosy, wondering why Jaz looked so triumphant. After all, it was *Rosy* who'd just single-brainedly solved the mystery of her Midnight Visitor.

'I figured out the next object!' announced Jaz, dropping onto Rosy's unmade bed and beaming at her.

'You mean – that yellow stone with the twig inside it?' said Rosy, diverted. 'Really? What is it?'

But Jaz was now staring at the desk. 'What's all that white stuff on your desk? Is that *flour*?'

'Oh, I thought I'd cleaned it all up,' said Rosy, glancing over. 'It didn't really work, anyway. At least, the camera did, but not in the way I'd planned. The tripwire was meant to turn on the camera, but she actually knocked it over and the noise woke me up.'

'Wait, is this your Midnight Visitor?' asked Jaz. 'Did you figure it out? Was it Ms Boydell?'

'Yes,' said Rosy. 'I mean, yes, I figured out the Midnight Visitor, but no, it wasn't Ms Boydell. I didn't think it could be, not once I realised ... But no, you started first. Go on.'

'No, *you*,' said Jaz, settling back on the bed. 'Come on, all of it! Background research, hypothesis, experimental procedure, the lot!'

'All right,' said Rosy happily, because she really *had* been longing to tell someone how clever she'd been. 'Wait, I need my notebook. Here it is, I wrote a summary.'

And she showed Jaz the relevant page, which said:

BACKGROUND OBSERVATIONS

Night 1 open window + apple –> papers on desk messed up + apple missing
Night 2 open window + no apple –> papers on desk NOT messed up

'So,' said Rosy, 'I decided the apple *had* to have something to do with my papers getting messed up. I mean, there were a whole lot of other things in my room as well, but they didn't change between Night 1 and Night 2. The only thing that was different was the apple being there or not there. That was the variable.'

'Okay,' said Jaz.

'But then, look at this,' said Rosy, and she pointed to the next line:

Night 3 open window + no apple –> papers on desk messed up

Chapter Seventeen

'Hmm,' said Jaz. 'I guess that's why scientists have to do their experiments more than once. Because sometimes things are just a coincidence. It looks like the apple had nothing to do with it, after all.'

'That's what I thought, too,' said Rosy. 'But then I did some closer observations. I looked at the bin that had been knocked over – the bin I hadn't emptied when I'd tidied my room earlier that night. And there was a banana peel in there – well, technically, half a banana peel. The other half was missing. There was a variable I'd overlooked! So I had to add that to my data.'

And she indicated the changes she'd made to her page:

Night 3 (revised data) open window + no apple + banana peel –> papers on desk messed up + half banana peel missing

'The door was locked each night,' Rosy went on, 'and after the first night, I put a chair in front of it so that if anyone had a key to unlock it and walked in, they'd have bumped into the chair and woken me up. There wasn't any other access to the room except through the open window. And now it seemed that fruit was involved in some way.'

'Hmm,' said Jaz, frowning.

'I thought it must be something coming in to eat the fruit. Maybe a flying fox? I know they're really fruit bats, not foxes, and you can hear them flapping around the trees here at sunset. So I asked the lady at the Macleay Museum and she said that although they *do* eat fruit, they prefer native fruit and flowers, and even then, they pick them off trees themselves. She didn't think it was very likely that one would fly through a window and scavenge for food inside a building. But then she said it could be a *possum*. They live in gum trees, they like fruit and they're not usually scared of people. So that was my hypothesis. I just had to figure out how to test it.'

She turned to the next page, which said:

EXPERIMENT

PHASE ONE

Night 4 closed window + no apple –> papers on desk NOT messed up

Night 5 closed window + apple –> papers on desk NOT messed up, apple NOT touched

Night 6 closed window + no apple –> papers on desk NOT messed up

'It does look as though whatever's messing up the papers was coming through the window,' said Jaz. 'But that doesn't prove it was a fruit-eating animal, let alone a possum.'

'That's why I moved on to Phase Two,' said Rosy. 'I wanted to find out if the papers had anything to do with it.'

PHASE TWO

Night 7 open window + apple on desk + all papers cleared off desk and stacked on bookshelf –> apple missing + papers on bookshelf NOT messed up

Chapter Seventeen

Night 8 open window + banana slices on desk + all papers cleared off desk and stacked on bookshelf
–> banana missing + papers on book-shelf NOT messed up

'So it seems the Midnight Visitor was more interested in fruit than my papers,' said Rosy. 'The papers probably got messed up accidentally when the Midnight Visitor was grabbing the fruit. Oh, and then Lynette told me there was a Vet Science student staying in here last term! Vet Science students like animals, right? So she probably wouldn't have reported a possum to the authorities if one came in and ate her snacks occasionally. I know that's not *definitive* evidence, but it's another hint, isn't it? Still, what I really needed was a photo or something like that.'

Rosy gestured at her desk.

'I thought flour sprinkled over the desk might pick up paw prints, then I could take a photo of them and ask the flying fox lady to identify the animal. Plus, I set up a wire across the windowsill and attached it to my camera switch, so it'd turn on if the wire was disturbed. Then I turned out all the lights and I sat up in bed and I waited. And waited and waited and waited. And then I fell asleep because I was pretty tired. And then ... CRASH!'

'And? What was it?'

'A huge fluffy grey possum, sitting there in the middle of my desk, holding a piece of apple in her front paws.' Rosy smiled, remembering. 'She must have knocked over the camera with her tail, because she looked around at it, then back at me, as if to say "Why did you leave *that* there?" And, Jaz, clinging to her back was a *baby* possum, peeking at me with its big brown eyes! It was the cutest thing ever. I wish I'd been able to reach my camera. The mother possum just stared at me a moment as she chewed away at the apple, then she wedged it in her mouth and squeezed back through the window, leaving flour smeared all over the place.'

'Huh,' said Jaz. 'Possums.'

'Possums.' Rosy nodded.

'You did some good logical reasoning there,' said Jaz, looking at Rosy's notes.

'I know,' said Rosy, feeling very pleased with herself. She was an artist, but she was *also* a scientist. She was a scientific artist! Or maybe even an artistic scientist. She wished she could tell her mother all about it, but she supposed that could get a bit complicated, what with Rosy having neglected to inform Alison that someone was invading her room at night in the first place. 'So, anyway,' Rosy said, 'tell me about the next object.'

'Oh, right!' said Jaz. 'Well, on the way home, I was looking at that photo of the yellow stone and wondering if it really *was* a stone, because you can't usually see inside stones, can you? But when I'd picked it up, it hadn't felt like plastic or glass, so what else could it be? I just couldn't figure it out. But then after dinner, Kirin decided to put on a DVD and she chose … *Jurassic Park*!' And Jaz gave Rosy an expectant look.

'Um …' said Rosy.

Chapter Seventeen

'You know,' said Jaz encouragingly. 'Amber!'

'Who?' said Rosy.

Jaz sighed. 'Remember how the scientists in *Jurassic Park* first got hold of the dinosaur DNA that let them make new dinosaurs?'

'No,' said Rosy, 'because I haven't seen *Jurassic Park*. I can't watch movies like that. They're way too scary for me. I'm very sensitive, you know.'

'What are you talking about? You watch movies about mummies and vampires and zombies!'

'Yeah, but only old black-and-white ones. And those are all made-up stories. Dinosaurs are *real*.' Rosy gave a shudder.

'You've got about the same chance of being attacked by a dinosaur as you have of being attacked by a mummy,' said Jaz, 'which is no chance at all. Dinosaurs lived in a completely different time to humans and – Oh, never mind that. All you need to know is that in the movie, they found an ancient mosquito enclosed in amber, which is fossilised tree resin, and the mosquito had dinosaur blood in its stomach, and that's how the scientists got their dinosaur DNA. Anyway, our object is the same yellowy-orange colour as amber and I found out a way to *prove* if it's amber or not. Come on, let's try it out!'

Jaz and Rosy ran to the common room, where Jaz unlocked the cabinet and removed the yellow blob.

'Watch this,' she said, and she rubbed the blob vigorously along the hem of her T-shirt. In the dimness of the curtained room, Rosy thought she saw sparks fly off. Then Jaz took a strip of tissue and held it over the blob. The tissue immediately stuck itself to the blob. 'Static electricity,' said Jaz, giving a satisfied nod. 'Did you know the ancient Greeks called amber *ēlektron* because it could develop a charge? And that's where we get the word "electricity".'

'Okay, then,' said Rosy. 'It's amber. So ... Dr Huxley thought that electricity was an important part of the history of medicine?'

'No,' said Jaz. 'Well, I guess hospitals do use all sorts of electrical machines, but no, I think he was more interested in what's *inside* the amber. It's not a twig with a little leaf attached – it's an insect. See, there's its body and there's the head. Here's a leg, and another leg, and that oval is a wing.'

Rosy turned on the lamp and held up the piece of amber, turning it sideways and upside down. 'Oh, yeah. Maybe a wasp? Or one of those flying ants –'

'It's a mosquito! Look at the head. It's got a long tube sticking out of it, like mosquitos use to suck blood.'

'What, you think Dr Huxley was a *Jurassic Park* fan? That this object represents DNA?'

'You can't *really* get DNA out of amber-preserved insects. Amber is millions of years old and DNA deteriorates pretty quickly. No, I think it's the mosquito he was interested in. I mean, which animal has killed the most humans throughout history?'

'Sharks?' guessed Rosy. 'No, crocodiles. Tigers. Rabid dogs.'

Chapter Seventeen

'No, mosquitos! Because they spread malaria.'

'Oh. What about fleas? Because they spread the plague?'

'But hardly anyone dies of the plague now, do they? And malaria's been around even longer than the plague. Remember Naomi saying that ancient Egyptians used to get malaria? And I looked it up in one of my books last night and malaria's had a *huge* effect on world history. Like, there was an epidemic of malaria in the fifth century that might have contributed to the collapse of the Roman Empire. And malaria was such a problem in Africa that the British gave up trying to colonise Africa and sent their convicts to Australia instead. Also, the construction of the Panama Canal had to be abandoned because workers kept getting sick with malaria, so there wasn't an easy way to get from the Atlantic Ocean to the Pacific until the twentieth century, when they'd finally worked out what caused malaria and how to prevent it. And also –'

'Okay, okay, malaria is very significant,' said Rosy. 'I suppose you've written a ten-page report on it already.'

'I did do some research,' said Jaz, putting the amber back on its blue velvet square and locking the cabinet. 'But it was very complicated and confusing. It's okay, though, because we've got an appointment at the School of Tropical Medicine at eleven o'clock with a malaria expert and he can answer our questions.'

Rosy gaped at Jaz. 'How did you manage to arrange *that* last night?'

'I didn't. Your mum did, this morning. He's a friend of hers.'

'What? She ... How did she even know that ... I mean, WHAT?'

'Oh, I saw her this morning in the foyer as she was leaving and I told her, so she rang him.' Jaz shrugged. 'Do you want to hear what I've learned about malaria so far?'

'Yeah, okay,' said Rosy, rather grumpily. As far as she could recall, her mum hadn't even bothered to say goodbye to her that morning. Rosy was beginning to wonder if Alison thought Jaz would make a better daughter than Rosy. 'Go on, then.'

'Well, there are a few different types of malaria, but they all involve fevers,' said Jaz, picking up her notebook. 'You go cold, then hot and sweaty, then that repeats over and over again. Your spleen swells up, your red blood cells get destroyed, and you get headaches and sore joints and vomiting and convulsions. It sounds awful.'

'Does it kill people?'

'At least half a million people die of it each year, maybe more, but mostly it just makes people really tired and weak and more likely to die of other diseases. Even with treatment, the symptoms can keep coming back. Plus, it can cause permanent brain damage, especially in children. Anyway, doctors worked out fairly early on that people got malaria if they lived near swamps, but they couldn't figure out if the disease was caused by the water or by bad air hovering above the water. That's why it's called malaria – *mala aria* is Italian for "bad air". In the 1600s, they realised that Peruvian bark – that's cinchona – cured malaria and by 1820, some French scientists called Pelletier and Caventou had isolated its active ingredient and called it quinine. But it was very expensive and it did have some serious side effects.'

'Such as?'

'Such as making people go deaf.'

'Yes, that is a fairly bad side effect.'

Jaz turned the page in her notebook. 'Meanwhile, scientists were still trying to figure out what caused the disease. In 1880, a French doctor called Alphonse Laveran discovered tiny parasites wriggling around inside the red blood cells of people with malaria and he found the parasites disappeared if the patient was given quinine. Then an Italian, Camillo Golgi, worked out that the fever happened when the parasite was released into the bloodstream and he and his colleagues discovered some different forms of the malaria parasite.'

'When you say "parasite", you don't mean "mosquito", do you? I mean, they weren't looking at little baby mosquitos in people's blood, were they?'

'No, it was a tiny animal called Plasmodium that lives inside mosquitos, the way the plague bacteria live inside fleas. But the scientists didn't know that yet. In the late 1890s, a British doctor working in India called Ronald Ross discovered Plasmodium inside an anopheles mosquito that had fed on a malaria patient. Then the Italian team proved that an infected anopheles mosquito could spread malaria among people by biting them.'

'Good work, scientists! And then they won the Nobel Prize. Well, three of them, at least.'

'Ross and Laveran did. Actually, Golgi did, too, but not for his malaria research. There was still lots of work to do, though. They had to figure out why some anopheles mosquitos spread the disease and others didn't. There was a theory that the dangerous mosquitos had more teeth.'

'Do mosquitos *have* teeth?'

'I don't think so,' said Jaz, 'but that's as far as I got with my reading.'

They spent some time preparing a list of questions, then set off early for their appointment with the malaria expert because they had a couple of deliveries to make first. The Macleay Museum was deserted, so they had to leave the flying fox lady's envelope propped up on the reception desk, but they found Naomi, as they'd expected, in the Nicholson Museum. She was dusting a display of little mummified crocodiles.

'You are cordially invited to the opening of the Huxley Bequest exhibition at New College,' Rosy told her, handing over one of the invitations she'd designed and printed the night before. 'And there *will* be cordial.'

'But also tea and coffee,' added Jaz hastily.

'And other refreshments,' said Rosy. 'Oh, and in case you don't speak French, this bit, *répondez s'il vous plaît*, means "please tell us if you're coming or not".'

Chapter Seventeen

'Is this the collection with the *wedjat*-eye amulet?' said Naomi. 'Oh, I'd love to have a look at it. Thank you. I'd be delighted to accept your invitation.'

'Excellent,' said Rosy. '*Au revoir*, then! That's French for "see you tomorrow at four o'clock"!'

Rosy had already given her mother an invitation to pass on to Marcus, so the girls proceeded directly to the School of Tropical Medicine, where Dr Kel Hudson was waiting for them in an extremely messy office. (Messiness, Rosy had decided, was one sure sign of a Serious Scientist. The surface of his desk alone probably held dozens of potential scientific discoveries.)

'Hello! Hello! Have a seat,' he cried, grabbing armfuls of what appeared to be a very long wedding veil off a sofa, turning around on the spot with his burden, then dumping it on the floor next to his desk. 'So, you're Alison's daughter!' he said to Rosy. 'Going to follow in her footsteps, then? Another scientist in the family?'

'Possibly.' Actually, Rosy hadn't yet decided whether she was going to be a famous artist, a writer, an actor or some combination of the three, but there was no reason why she couldn't be scientific while she was doing any of them. 'And Jaz wants to be a doctor, don't you?'

'Or a medical researcher,' said Jaz, which was news to Rosy, although not very surprising news.

'Excellent,' said Dr Hudson, beaming at Jaz. 'Don't let Alison Radford talk you into working on boring old bacteria, though. Protozoa, that's where all the exciting stuff is happening!'

'Protozoa?' said Jaz. 'Is that what Plasmodium is, a type of protozoa?'

'Yes, and it's a sneaky little devil, considering it's only got one cell and no brain. *Plasmodium falciparum*, that's the one that causes the worst type of malaria. You know they get into people through the bite of an infected mosquito? But then those dastardly parasites hide out in the liver, away from the immune system, multiplying like crazy, until *boom*! They break out, disguised as liver cells, zoom into the bloodstream and start invading red blood cells. Then they multiply *again* inside the blood cells, the blood cells burst open, releasing more parasites into the blood, and the whole thing happens again and again. Not only that, they manage to stick all sorts of proteins on the outside of the blood cells, which makes it harder for the spleen to destroy the infection.'

'But some people are born resistant to malaria, aren't they?' said Jaz, consulting her notes.

'Hmm, yes and no,' he said. 'About a third of Africans and quite a lot of people in Saudi Arabia and India are born with the sickle-cell gene, which affects their red blood cells. If they only inherit one of those genes, they can still get malaria, but they probably won't get very sick from it. The problem is, if they have two of those genes, one from each parent, they're born with sickle-cell anaemia, which is a nasty disease in itself. Then there are the G6PD deficiency diseases, also genetic, common in men from Africa, the Middle East and South Asia. It protects them from

Chapter Seventeen

Plasmodium falciparum, but it causes anaemia under certain conditions – if they get an infection, if they take certain drugs or if they eat certain foods, such as broad beans. So … it's complicated.'

'But there are medicines to treat malaria now, right?' said Rosy. 'I mean, I know quinine had bad side effects, but scientists came up with new drugs, didn't they?'

'Yep, chloroquine was the first synthetic malaria drug, invented in the 1930s. Then there was another drug that was tested here in Australia during the Second World War, using volunteers. It seemed to work perfectly, so the army gave it to thousands of Allied soldiers fighting in New Guinea and what do you know, none of them got malaria! For a few months. But then they started collapsing with fevers. The army generals and doctors decided the soldiers must not be taking their tablets properly and made each man line up every day to have a tablet stuck in his mouth by an officer. But they *still* got sick. How could this be happening?'

'Resistance!' said Rosy. 'The parasite became resistant to the medicine.'

'Ah, I can tell you're a Radford,' said Dr Hudson, waggling his finger at her. 'Yes, Plasmodium became resistant to not just chloroquine, but practically any new drug we could invent. Fortunately, some Chinese scientists started researching traditional remedies and came up with artemisinin, made from sweet wormwood shrubs, and that worked really well. Eventually some strains of Plasmodium became resistant to that, too, but it's still our best treatment if it's used in combination with other drugs. The problem isn't just drug resistance, though. It's that most of the countries where people are dying of malaria also happen to be developing countries with hardly any money for medical staff or treatment clinics or testing labs.'

'What about preventing malaria?' said Jaz. 'Like, stopping mosquitos from biting people? That must be cheaper than building clinics and training doctors.'

'Ah, yes.' He waved his hand at the pile of white netting he'd dumped beside his desk. 'I've just got back from a conference about that. Mosquito nets treated with insecticides and hung over beds at night. Go to any anti-malaria charity website and you'll find lots of snazzy graphs showing the millions of nets that have been distributed to African families. But you know what?' He leaned in and lowered his voice. 'We're lucky if even half those nets get used effectively. People wash them, then they don't reapply the insecticide. They take them down in hot weather because it's too stuffy to sleep under a net. They turn them into wedding dresses or fishing nets. In some places, they're convinced the nets kill children and make women infertile, so they refuse to hang them over their beds. Lots of people don't even accept that mosquitos cause malaria. They believe it's the result of evil spirits or dirty water or bad weather. Oh, and anopheles mosquitos quickly become resistant to those insecticides, anyway.'

Chapter Seventeen

'Why doesn't the World Health Organization have a big campaign to eradicate malaria, like they're doing with polio?' asked Rosy.

'Well, there *was* a WHO campaign. It started in 1955 and was meant to wipe out malaria within ten years, but they'd given up by 1969. Malaria is ... Did I mention it was complicated? I actually meant to say that it's very, *very* complicated. There's no vaccine, for one thing, and I can't see one being developed any time soon. There are at least five different species of Plasmodium that can cause malaria in humans, each one with multiple stages of development. It's spread by dozens of species of mosquitos and it can survive in lots of other animals. How do you come up with an effective weapon against that? Killing mosquitos did seem the best thing to do and for a while, they had success using a powerful insecticide called DDT. Problem is, DDT doesn't just kill mosquitos. It has an effect on other insects, on fish, on birds – which is why it got banned in the United States in 1972. And there were all sorts of unexpected consequences of killing mosquitos. You've heard the story of the parachuting cats?'

'Parachuting *cats*?' said Rosy, picturing her neighbour's tabby kitten in flying goggles and a little harness, drifting down to earth under a handkerchief-sized canopy.

'Oh, you'll like this one!' Dr Hudson rubbed his hands. 'Well, in Borneo in the 1950s, the WHO anti-malaria teams sprayed people's huts with insecticide and it did get rid of the mosquitos. Unfortunately, it also killed a type of wasp that killed caterpillars, so there were lots more caterpillars, which ate the thatched roofs of the huts, which then collapsed on top of the people who lived in the huts.

'Not only that, their cats started dying. Either the cats were eating poisoned insects and lizards or they were licking insecticide off their own fur, but regardless, the cat population went down and the rat population went up. Of course, rats can spread diseases that are just as bad as malaria – plague, for instance – so something had to be done. The villages needed more cats, pronto! The problem was, a lot of these villages were very isolated, in the mountains, with no roads, so the solution was to collect cats from the coastal towns, then parachute them in. Not with their own individual parachutes, of course, but in special cat baskets, dropped by the air force. And the cats arrived safely and ate the rats and that was that!

'But it just goes to show how tricky it is, trying to make things better. You never know what the consequences will be. Now the WHO has started up another campaign, but this time it's trying to *control* malaria, not wipe it out completely, and they've stopped thinking there'll ever be an easy fix for the problem. Each community has its own set of unique issues and locals often have a better idea of what will work than do people like me, sitting in our offices on the other side of the world. Oh, and by the way, the WHO has gone back to recommending the use of DDT now.'

Chapter Seventeen

'But don't the mosquitos become resistant to that, as well?' asked Jaz.

'Oh, yes,' said Dr Hudson. 'And people keep cutting down forests for mining and agriculture, exposing themselves to brand new species of parasite. A few years ago, we found malaria patients in Malaysia infected with a species of Plasmodium that we only used to find in monkeys. And with climate change, there'll be hotter temperatures and more rain – even better conditions for mosquitos to thrive. Oh, the fight against malaria is only just beginning!'

He looked quite cheerful about it, Rosy observed. But then, she supposed he didn't have to worry about ever being out of a job.

CHAPTER EIGHTEEN

You're qualified. But we've never had a woman in the laboratory before, and we think you'd be a distracting influence.'
~ Gertrude B. Elion

On the way back to New College, Jaz came to a sudden halt in the middle of the road and stared up at the School of Physics.

'Those names along the top of the building,' she said. 'Have they always been there?'

'No, a team of possums chiselled them into the sandstone while we were talking to Dr Hudson,' said Rosy. 'Of *course* they've always been there. You'd have noticed them before if you didn't walk about all the time with your nose in a book.'

Jaz chose to ignore this. 'KEPLER,' she read aloud. 'GALILEO. NEWTON ... Hmm, what's that one meant to be? Oh, they're using a V instead of a U again. FOURIER. I think he was a mathematician.'

'Did any of them have any connection whatsoever to the history of medicine?' asked Rosy, without much hope. After all, what did physics have to do with medicine? Not that Rosy was entirely sure what physics *was*. Electricity, magnets, atoms, that sort of thing?

'ROENTGEN,' said Jaz, who'd reached the end of the building. 'That sounds familiar. I'm sure it was in one of my medical history books ... Now, *where* did I see it?'

While Jaz was pondering this, Rosy had the bright idea of visiting the School of Medicine. 'Maybe that has names carved on it, too,' she said. 'It might give us some clues for Dr Huxley's last object – you know, the metal spiral.'

'But we've already looked at that building, haven't we?' said Jaz. 'Isn't it the one with the statues of Harvey and Pasteur in front?'

'No, that's the New Medical School,' said Rosy. 'Well, New-ish. The original building is from the 1800s. It's across the road from the Nicholson Museum.'

So they turned and headed back up the hill. A pair of cherubs over the entranceway of the imposing sandstone building held up an elaborate scroll announcing that this was indeed the 'FACULTY OF MEDICINE', although there didn't seem to be any names carved anywhere.

'Perhaps they've got some statues or portraits inside,' said Jaz, but when they tried the front door, it refused to budge.

'Locked out,' said Rosy, shaking her head. 'And you know why, don't you? It's because we're *girls*.'

'Well, I think it's just locked because it's the summer holidays ...'

Chapter Eighteen

'No,' said Rosy firmly, as they turned back. 'It's *symbolic*. Did you know that the first woman medical student to enrol here wasn't allowed to pass her final exams, because the head of the medical school reckoned that a woman's proper place was in the home? And they named this *building* after him, but *she* had to travel all the way to England to do her exams before she could become a doctor. Mum told me about it. Oh, and there was something else I read! At the University of Edinburgh, there was actually a *riot* in 1870 about the first women medical students. The male students were furious because one of the women came first in their exam and won a scholarship. Not that the university actually gave her the scholarship – they gave it to a man who'd got a lower mark.'

'That's so unfair!'

'I know, and then it went to court and the judge said women shouldn't have been allowed to enrol in the first place. But listen, one of the women, Sophia Jex-Blake, decided if they weren't going to let women study medicine, then she'd set up her *own* medical school for women. So she did, in London, and guess who helped her? Thomas Huxley! Oh, and there was another woman in America who won a medal for being an army surgeon in the Civil War, but they took away her medal because she stopped wearing corsets and started campaigning for women to be allowed to vote …'

The girls paused outside Mohammad's booth to hand over his invitation. Jaz had raised mild objections to this, but Rosy had pointed out that people coming to the party might want to park their cars outside the college and it would be good if Mohammad was inside having cordial and chips, rather than outside, sticking parking tickets on people's cars. Anyway, he *had* told them about Arabic medicine and he *was* about to become a medical student. Probably.

And he sounded keen when Rosy explained about Dr Huxley's bequest, although he said he'd have to double-check his work schedule. Then Rosy and Jaz went up to the common room to inspect the thirteenth and final object: the metal spiral. They had twenty-four hours to figure it out.

'What do you think it's made from?' said Rosy, weighing it in one hand. 'Silver? Platinum?'

'Aluminium,' said Jaz. 'It's some sort of spring, isn't it? Look, you can squash it down. Maybe it's part of a medical machine.'

'No, I reckon it's *symbolic*,' said Rosy. 'Like, a model of something. Hey! What about DNA? You know how people say DNA is a double helix? "Helix" is just a fancy way of saying "spiral", isn't it? And DNA is part of the history of medicine.'

'But a double helix means there'd have to be two spirals,' said Jaz. 'No, I think this object's more likely to be from some sort of technology. It looks so shiny and modern compared to all the other things in the cabinet. Let's go and do some research. I want to look up Roentgen, anyway, before I forget.'

In Rosy's room, Jaz commandeered Methuselah and quickly found what she was looking for. 'Roentgen took the first X-ray photo,' she reported. 'Look, here's his X-ray of his wife's hand from 1895, showing all her finger bones and the rings she was wearing. When she saw it, she said, "I have seen my death!"'

'I thought Marie Curie was the one who discovered X-rays,' said Rosy.

'No, she was the one who discovered radiation. No, wait – Henri Becquerel found that uranium gave off strange rays, but Marie Curie worked out it was because the uranium atom was emitting radiation, and then she and her husband, Pierre, discovered two new radioactive elements, polonium and radium. She's the only person to have won Nobel Prizes for both Physics and Chemistry. Her daughter Irène won a Nobel Prize for her work on radioactivity, too. Not that either of them could join the French Academy of Sciences. No women allowed till 1962.'

'Typical,' huffed Rosy. 'Hey, and did you notice the name CURIE written anywhere on that Physics building? No!'

'Well, maybe it was hidden behind those trees at the end of the building ... Oh, look, this is really sad. In 1934, Marie Curie died of aplastic anaemia caused by all the radiation she worked with. Even now, her papers are so radioactive that anyone wanting to look at them has to wear special protective clothing. I guess back then, people just didn't understand how dangerous radiation was. They actually sold radioactive "health drinks" in the 1920s! And shoe shops used to X-ray children's feet just to make sure their shoes fitted.'

'But radiation does good as well as harm,' Rosy said. 'I mean, how did they work out if you had broken bones or big holes in your teeth before X-rays were invented?'

'I know,' said Jaz. 'And they've got CT scans now, as well, which are even more powerful and can look at your brain and all your internal organs. And doctors can use radiation to kill cancer cells. But that's the problem – the radiation can damage normal cells as well. It says here that some cancers are actually *caused* by CT scans. And then when patients have radiotherapy to cure their cancer, all that extra radiation can cause *new* cancer.'

'Wait,' said Rosy, suddenly worried. 'What about ultrasounds? Are they dangerous, too? Because Gabrielle had some of them when she was pregnant, to see if Reuben was growing okay.'

'No, it says ultrasounds are much safer,' said Jaz, studying the screen. 'They're not radioactive, they're just sound waves. There are MRI scans, too, which use magnetic fields, although you can't have one of those if you've got any metal inside your body.'

It was amazing, really, all the different helpful machines that science had invented, although Rosy remained unconvinced that the thirteenth object represented medical technology. She thought it far more likely that Dr Huxley would have included DNA in his collection. But when she said this to Jaz, Jaz just set her jaw in that way she had and went on doggedly typing up her notes about medical imaging technology. Jaz was so *stubborn*, thought Rosy.

Chapter Eighteen

So she waited till Jaz had gone home for the day, then spent the entire evening trying to find out what DNA actually was. This proved to be rather complicated, so it was lucky she had her mother sitting at the other end of the table, tapping away at her own laptop. Rosy was used to working alongside her dad in his studio, sharing paintbrushes and gluepots and offering each other helpful feedback on their progressing artworks, but it was nice to be able to share something with her mum for once.

'Right, I think I've got it now,' said Rosy at last. 'So, human bodies are made up of millions of cells and most of those cells contain DNA, which basically means a long line of genes. And each little gene carries a code that tells the body how it should look or how to do important stuff. Like, a gene might say whether you have brown eyes or blue eyes, or whether drinking cow's milk will make you feel sick. And each person gets half their DNA from their dad and half from their mum, but sometimes when the DNA is copying itself to make new cells, it can make mistakes and that can cause genetic diseases. Right? Right. No, wait, what's a chromosome? Is it these worm-looking things in the middle of each cell?'

Alison peered over. 'Yep. A chromosome is just DNA in a double helix shape, coiled around some proteins. Humans have twenty-two pairs of chromosomes in each cell, plus usually either an X and a Y chromosome, if they're male, or two X chromosomes, if they're female.'

'A double helix,' repeated Rosy thoughtfully, looking at her sketches. 'That's this thing that looks like a ladder twisted round and round.'

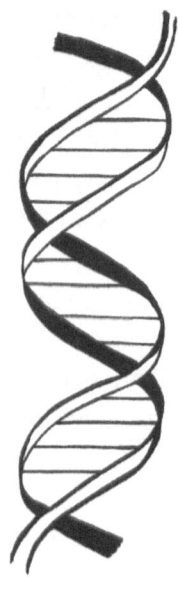

It didn't resemble Dr Huxley's metal spiral in the slightest, but Rosy decided to find out who had discovered the double helix shape of DNA, anyway. Ten minutes later, she gave a squawk of indignation.

'Mum!' Rosy cried. 'Did you realise that Francis Crick and James Watson took Rosalind Franklin's research data without asking her and used it to figure out that DNA was a double helix in 1953 and then they didn't acknowledge her work when they published their research and *then* they got the Nobel Prize and they didn't even mention her name in their speech! And then Watson wrote a book saying Rosalind Franklin was too stupid to understand her own data! Even though she was actually amazingly clever and did loads of important work on DNA and viruses!'

'Of course I know about Rosalind Franklin,' said Alison. 'Why else would I have named you after her?'

Rosy gaped at her mother. 'What?' she exclaimed. 'No, you didn't! I was named after Rosalind Atkins, the artist! Remember, you were pregnant with me and you and Dad went to see an exhibition of her engravings and I kept kicking whenever you stopped to look at one of the prints.'

Chapter Eighteen

'Oh, well, yes, there was that,' acknowledged Alison. 'And your father was determined to name you after an artist. But *I* wanted to name you after a scientist, so that's how you ended up as Rosalind.'

'You named me after *Rosalind Franklin*?' said Rosy. 'Someone who wasn't even allowed in the common room of the college where she did her research because she was a woman, someone who got cheated out of a Nobel Prize?'

'I named you after a brave, beautiful woman of great integrity and intelligence, who refused to let anyone distract her from her work,' said Alison. 'Now, didn't I choose well?'

'Hmph,' said Rosy, but she felt herself grow warm with pleasure. She busied herself with Methuselah for a while. 'Well, they did eventually name a building after her at Cambridge University,' said Rosy at last. 'As well as a lab at the University of London. And a medical school in America.'

She glanced at her mother, who was tapping away at her laptop again. Rosy's thoughts turned to Jaz and her career plans. Jaz was super smart and *extremely* stubborn, but still …

'Hey, Mum?' Rosy said. 'Is it very difficult, being a woman scientist? These days, I mean.'

Alison considered. 'Yes,' she said after a moment. 'Sometimes. But then, it's difficult being a *scientist*. Experiments that take months to set up and don't produce any results, lab equipment breaking down at a crucial point, research funds running out, having to spend hours doing pointless paperwork to keep university administrators happy. But when you discover something new and exciting, when you know your work will save lives and make the world a better place …' She smiled. 'It's worth it. Most of the really valuable, meaningful things in life take a lot of time and effort. *You* know that.'

Rosy thought of her very best painting, which had won second prize in the National Student Art Competition and had taken her nearly a year to finish, and she nodded. Then she looked back down at her notes. 'What about discovering DNA?' she asked. 'Was *that* worthwhile? I mean, did it save lives? Did it make the world a better place?'

'Good question,' said Alison. 'Well, we now know a lot about human genes and what they do. That means we can look at a person's DNA and make predictions about their health. Is that useful? It depends. For example, you might have a gene that suggests you're more likely to develop heart disease. So you can stop smoking, change your diet, do more exercise, maybe take medicine to lower your blood pressure or your cholesterol – but you can do that anyway, whether you have that gene or not, and it'll greatly reduce your risk of dying of a heart attack. And what if it's a disease, a serious one, that can't be prevented? How would it help someone to know they're likely to develop a debilitating illness that will probably kill them, when there's nothing they can do to stop it?'

As Rosy was pondering this, Alison added, 'Remember, no medical test is one hundred per cent accurate. Some genetic tests aren't very reliable at all.

Chapter Eighteen

There are a few American companies that offer genetic tests over the internet and when investigators sent four of them the same DNA sample, each company came up with a completely different health prediction. Anyway, no genetic test can say for certain what will happen for the rest of your life, because your health is affected by a lot of things other than genes.'

'Oh,' said Rosy. Then she remembered something. 'Hey, you know when Gabrielle was pregnant with Reuben? She had a genetic test to see if he might have Down Syndrome, because the doctor said she should. But afterwards, she said she didn't know what she'd have done if the test said he *did* have it. Probably nothing, she reckoned. Her friend Sarah's little boy has Down Syndrome and he's lovely. Much less violent than Reuben, anyway.'

'Well, there are a lot of challenges bringing up a child who has disabilities, but plenty of parents manage it and wouldn't change their child for anything. People need to decide for themselves whether a disease or a disability is so severe that it's worth testing for. There are a lot of ethical issues raised by DNA technology.'

Rosy was now certain that DNA was important enough to make it into Dr Huxley's collection, although the more she looked at her photo of the metal spiral, the less it resembled a double helix. But what else could it represent? She decided to ask her mum what *she* believed was the most important medical discovery of the last fifty years.

'Most important? You mean, the most helpful?' Alison looked thoughtful. 'Well, there've been a lot of discoveries about our immune system, so now we can treat diseases more effectively and stop people dying from allergic reactions. It also means we can transplant organs like kidneys and lungs into patients without their bodies rejecting them. There have been significant advances in mental health, too – we're better at helping people with depression and schizophrenia and so on. But if I had to choose just one, it'd probably be finding out that smoking kills people. Quit-smoking campaigns have probably saved more lives than anything else. Although, as a *scientist*, I'd be tempted to say it was developing tissue culture techniques, so we can grow live cells in a lab for research …'

Hopeless. None of them had anything to do with metal spirals. But it did give Rosy an idea.

CHAPTER NINETEEN

'It is a good morning exercise for a research scientist to discard a pet hypothesis every day before breakfast. It keeps him young.'
~ Konrad Lorenz

Jaz was very interested in Rosy's DNA research when Rosy told her about it the next morning.

'Oh, you're right,' Jaz said. 'Genetic testing *is* really important.' She peered at the metal spiral in the cabinet. 'Maybe more important than medical imaging machines …'

'Yeah, but, Jaz, I was thinking,' said Rosy, 'maybe genetic tests aren't so great. I mean, what if they told you that you were going to get some incurable fatal disease?'

'I'd want to know anyway,' said Jaz at once.

'But would you *really*?' asked Rosy. 'You might start thinking there was no point to anything. You might take lots of dangerous risks, if you were convinced you were going to die.'

'We're all going to die.'

'I know, but most people die when they're *old*. It'd be really depressing to know you were going to die young.'

'It'd be more depressing to die young and not be prepared for it.'

'But –'

'You don't know anything about it,' said Jaz obstinately, starting to glower at Rosy. So Rosy quickly told Jaz about Rosalind Franklin getting cheated out of a Nobel Prize and Jaz directed her irritation at Watson and Crick and the Nobel Prize committee, which was much better, from Rosy's perspective. The two girls were well into a big grumble about the topic when Alison popped in to let them know she was off to her lab.

'Have *you* ever met a Nobel Prize winner, Dr Radford?' asked Jaz.

'Oh, yes,' said Alison. 'You run into lots of interesting people at scientific conferences. I met Elizabeth Blackburn a couple of years ago at one of those Women in Science things – fascinating research she's doing in genetics. Not really my area, but quite intriguing, and she was born in Australia, too. Oh, and I know Barry, of course. Barry and Robin. Rosy, *you've* met Barry.'

'Barry? Barry who?'

'Barry Marshall. I knew him and Robin Warren years ago, when I was working in Perth. Then I happened to catch the same flight as him not long after they'd both won the Nobel and you and your father came to pick me up from the airport that night.'

'I don't remember this at all,' said Rosy.

'Well, you were only four or five. Everyone thought you were adorable. You had on your pyjamas and your little furry slippers.'

Chapter Nineteen

'Pyjamas!'

'Yes, your cowgirl ones. You'd insisted on wearing your cowgirl hat, too.'

'This is absolutely *mortifying*,' Rosy said to Jaz. 'I get to meet a Nobel Prize winner and not only do I forget all about it afterwards, but I'm told I was wearing *cowgirl pyjamas* at the time.'

Jaz managed to stop laughing long enough to ask Alison why the two men had won the Nobel Prize.

'Oh, they were very clever,' said Alison. 'They found a new species of bacteria living in human stomachs and worked out it could cause stomach problems, including ulcers. Until then, doctors thought that ulcers were caused by stress or spicy foods, so they treated ulcers with medicine that decreased acid in the stomach. The problem was that the ulcers tended to come back as soon as the patient stopped taking the medicine. After Barry and Robin's discovery, doctors realised they could give antibiotics to kill the bacteria and that was a much more effective and long-lasting cure.'

'That was a very *useful* discovery,' said Jaz approvingly.

'Yes, and they had a bit of luck finding the bacteria in the first place, because *Helicobacter pylori* is very tricky to see, let alone grow in pure cultures. But they were persistent, too, and passionate about what they were doing. It was quite difficult to test their hypothesis, because *H. pylori* can't survive very well in animals other than humans. They tried experimenting on pigs, but that didn't work. So Barry drank some of the bacteria to see what would happen to his own stomach.'

'What?' cried Rosy and Jaz.

'Oh, don't worry,' Alison assured them, 'it worked. He developed all the symptoms of gastric disease. Then he got a doctor to look inside his stomach with an endoscope and take samples of his stomach lining for testing and it all supported their hypothesis.'

'Wait,' said Rosy. 'Back up a bit. He drank *dangerous bacteria*?'

'Well, it wasn't that dangerous,' said Alison. 'I mean, there was already a treatment for stomach ulcers. And Barry's wife made him take antibiotics afterwards and he was fine.'

Rosy and Jaz exchanged a long look.

'*You* wouldn't experiment on yourself like that, would you?' Rosy asked her mother.

'Oh, no,' said Alison. 'Well, probably not. I mean, only if there weren't any other alternatives ...'

After she'd left, Rosy turned to Jaz. 'Are you *sure* you want to be a medical researcher?' Rosy asked.

'Maybe I could research something other than bacteria,' said Jaz, who was now looking a bit worried.

Then they both remembered they were supposed to be figuring out the metal spiral and Rosy recalled the idea she'd had the previous night.

'Let's do a survey of everyone we can find, asking them what *they* think is the most important discovery in modern medicine. Then maybe one of those ideas will have something to do with metal spirals.'

Chapter Nineteen

The first person they encountered was a young man perched on top of a ladder in the middle of the corridor, fiddling with the light fitting on the ceiling.

'G'day,' he said when he saw them. 'Do us a favour and pass up that light bulb, would you?'

For safety's sake, they waited till he'd finished screwing in the bulb and had climbed down before asking if he'd participate in their survey.

'It's only one question and we won't write down your name or anything, so it's anonymous,' said Rosy. 'What do you think is the most important medical advance of the past fifty years?'

He contemplated this as he wiped his hands on a rag. 'What, you mean, my personal opinion? Well ... I reckon antiretroviral drugs to fight AIDS. Yeah, there are a lot of HIV-positive people around these days who are alive and healthy, thanks to those drugs. Including me.'

'Oh, that's a good answer!' said Rosy. 'We hadn't thought of that one.'

'Rosy,' chided Jaz. 'You're not supposed to say anything to our survey participants apart from the question, in case you bias the results. It *is* a good answer, though,' she told the electrician.

'Cheers,' he said, grinning. 'What's this survey for, anyway? School? They're not making you do homework in the holidays, are they?'

'This is *much* more interesting than school,' said Rosy. 'Are you going to be working here for the rest of the day?' He nodded. 'Well, come to the Senior

Common Room at four o'clock. The College is celebrating its new collection of artefacts about the history of medicine and you're cordially invited.'

She handed him an invitation, then she and Jaz proceeded downstairs to the office to survey Lynette, who immediately said, 'The Pill.'

'What pill?' said Rosy.

'Birth control pills,' said Lynette. 'You girls have no idea what it used to be like. But suddenly women could *choose* when to have a baby or whether to have one at all. Oh, it was wonderful! The Pill changed our lives.'

Then Ms Boydell walked in with Dr Adam, the Master of the College. Dr Adam, recently returned from a holiday on the Gold Coast, nominated CPR – cardiopulmonary resuscitation – because he'd watched some surf lifesavers revive a drowned man on the beach. 'They used those electric paddles to restart his heart,' Dr Adam recalled. 'Miraculous stuff!'

Ms Boydell said it was medical researchers figuring out what caused Sudden Infant Death Syndrome and then telling everyone that babies should sleep on their backs, not their stomachs. 'My sister's first baby died of SIDS,' she said, 'and it was terrible. I'd never want any other mother to go through what she did and now there's a way to prevent it, thanks to science.' Lynette put a sympathetic arm around Ms Boydell's shoulders.

Then Mrs Adam walked in and she said chemotherapy, which had saved her father's life when he had cancer, and Dr Adam started patting *her* on the back.

Chapter Nineteen

The grown-ups were all getting a bit emotional, so Rosy and Jaz made a hasty escape. They found Ferdinand in the cleaner's cupboard and he said insulin injections to treat diabetes, although Jaz later checked in one of her books and found insulin had been discovered in 1921, which was not exactly recent. Ferdinand's wife, Emmy, chose the internet, because she said she used it all the time, to look up her symptoms whenever she was sick.

'Yes, you have a little bit of a headache and then you go online and decide it's a brain tumour,' said Ferdinand, rolling his eyes.

'The internet is very important to medicine,' said Emmy firmly. 'Even doctors use it to share information. Even *scientists* use it.' She pointed her mop at Jaz. 'Write it down.'

They left Ferdinand and Emmy arguing in the cupboard and went down to the kitchen. Maurice, the cook, said it was people being made to wear seatbelts in cars now and random breath testing to stop drunk drivers. Jaz raised her eyebrows at Rosy to say, *Is that really a <u>medical</u> advance or a legal one?* and Rosy quickly eyebrowed back, *Yes, it's medical, because it saves lives, and don't argue with him because he said he'd bake us some sausage rolls for the party this afternoon.*

Then the man who was delivering a box of vegetables nominated the Bionic Ear, an electronic implant that helped deaf people hear, and the two dentistry students they found in the foyer said it was putting fluoride in the water supply to stop everyone's teeth rotting.

Rosy wanted to survey Jaz's dad as well, but Jaz said they couldn't disturb him because he was busy working.

'He's coming to the party, though, right?' said Rosy.

'Yes, and that's why he's so busy now. He has to get all those plants into the side garden before then.'

Rosy started to ask how one little question would delay his work when she was distracted by the sky. 'Hey – isn't that a cloud?'

'Oh, yeah!' said Jaz, gazing upwards. 'They did say on the news that there might be a cool change this weekend. Look, there's another one. It's a bit grey, too!'

Energised by the thought of a break in the weather, they rushed off to Alison's flat to study their survey results. The problem was that none of these recent medical advances seemed to have much to do with metal spirals.

'Right,' Jaz said grimly, after they'd been debating the issue for nearly half an hour. 'Let's just say it's part of an X-ray machine.' She reached for Methuselah.

'We can't do that!' Rosy protested. 'We don't have any evidence for that at all.'

'So?' said Jaz. 'Who's going to know?'

Rosy yanked Methuselah away from her. 'It doesn't matter whether they know,' said Rosy sternly. *'We'll* know. It's … it's scientific fraud! Do you want to be like William McBride, making up stuff to suit your hypothesis?'

'No.' Jaz looked abashed.

Chapter Nineteen

'No, neither do I,' said Rosy. 'So let's do what a proper scientist does. Let's write that we don't know what it is, but we have some hypotheses. And then we can put up a list of everyone's anonymous survey answers. And ... I know, we can leave space for people to write more ideas below that!'

The rest of the afternoon vanished in a blur of activity. They laminated and pinned up the last pages of their research on the noticeboard beside the cabinet. Then they covered the big table in the common room with a white linen cloth and set out plates of chocolate-chip cookies and caramel brownies and salt-and-vinegar chips, and made little labels listing the ingredients for all the food, in case anyone was allergic, and lugged towers of coffee cups and glasses and an esky full of ice up the stairs from the kitchen. It was hot, tiring work, but each time they glanced out the window, more and more of the sky was streaked with cloud and a breeze was beginning to rattle the palm trees in the courtyard.

'Might even have a storm tonight,' observed Lynette, when she came in to switch on the coffee machine. 'Oh, this is *very* impressive!' She was looking at Dr Huxley's collection of objects, all neatly arranged behind freshly polished glass.

'Do you think the lawyer will be satisfied with it?' asked Jaz.

'Let's hope so,' said Lynette fervently. 'Because we've already spent all that money in our heads. Be a shame if we can't actually carry out our grand plans, won't it? Ooh, but I'd better get back down to the office, in case he's arrived.'

She hurried off, just as the other invited guests began to drift in. First was Rosy's mum, direct from the lab, her satchel still slung over her shoulder, accompanied by Marcus, whose T-shirt said, 'MICROBIOLOGY: ALL THE COOL KIDS ARE DOING IT!' Alison took him straight over to the cabinet to show him Alexander Fleming's mould.

They were joined by Dr Bennet, who pointed at Lind's scurvy pages with her walking stick and proudly announced that she'd been the one who'd deciphered them. Then Dr Hudson, the malaria expert, helped Maurice carry in the trays of little quiches and sausage rolls – it turned out the two men were old mates who played in the same university rugby team each winter.

The flying fox lady arrived, deep in a discussion with the electrician, who wanted to know how to stop flying foxes electrocuting themselves on overhead wires, followed by Naomi, looking very pretty in a flowered sundress. Then Rosy caught sight of Mohammad hovering shyly in the doorway, so she dragged him over to talk to Jaz's dad, who was listening with interest to Dr Hudson's account of his recent trip to India.

Everyone found the artefacts fascinating. They gathered round the cabinet, saying things like 'What on earth is *that*?' and 'Well, I never!' and then feeling their heads for bumps and consulting the phrenological head and snorting with laughter. Naomi was bombarded with questions about ancient Egyptian medicine, then

Chapter Nineteen

people turned on Dr Hudson to interrogate him about the history of malaria.

'Although really, you should be addressing all your questions to these two young ladies,' he said, indicating Rosy and Jaz. 'Remarkably well informed about all manner of things medical and historical –'

But the crowd suddenly fell silent, for there in the doorway stood Dr Adam and a tall, besuited stranger.

'Well!' Dr Adam said, rather nervously. 'Ahem. As you can see, the college very much appreciates Dr Huxley's bequest. Such intriguing objects! On display, of course, as requested, but securely locked away behind that glass. I do hope it meets the requirements of ... er ...'

The crowd hastily parted to clear a path to the cabinet, which the stranger was stalking towards with an expression of great intensity. Dr Adam trailed behind, accompanied by Lynette and Ms Boydell, the three of them wearing identical apprehensive expressions. Now the man was examining the contents of the cabinet, then turning to stare at the accompanying notes. Everyone in the room seemed to have stopped breathing. Rosy reached out for Jaz's wrist and squeezed it. Then the man whirled around and Rosy saw with horror that his face was mottled, his eyes blinking rapidly.

'This,' the man said, pointing to the notes. 'Who did all this?'

Rosy took a reluctant step forward. Jaz, still attached to Rosy by the wrist, came with her.

'We did,' they said as one. Then, slightly louder, Rosy said, 'We did it. We did all of it.'

'Oh,' said the man. 'Oh – he would have *loved* this!' And with a few strides, he was in front of Rosy and Jaz and wringing each of their hands in turn. 'It's marvellous! Quite marvellous!'

And everybody else burst into applause. Dr Adam's shoulders slumped with relief and Lynette and Ms Boydell gave each other a surreptitious high five.

'He had such a passion for education,' the man was saying to Rosy and Jaz. 'For learning, for science –' He broke off, produced a large polka-dotted handkerchief and blew his nose. 'Forgive me. I do miss him. Oh, and I haven't even introduced myself! Rufus Huxley, solicitor. He was my great uncle, you know. I don't usually deal with wills and such, but he insisted I be the executor of his estate … Anyway, you must tell me *all* you've discovered. I remember when he acquired the Egyptian amulet and Fleming's medallion – oh, he was tremendously excited about that medallion, apparently Fleming used to give them out to visiting dignitaries, even the royal family. But the significance of some of these objects is a complete mystery to me.'

They went over to the cabinet and Rosy and Jaz began explaining about the objects, although the girls had as many questions for him as he had for them.

'Are you related to Thomas Huxley?' asked Rosy. 'The famous one?'

'Oh, very distantly,' said the younger Huxley. 'Third cousin, twice removed or some such thing. Uncle Timothy was quite proud of the connection, though.'

Chapter Nineteen

'And was he a doctor?' said Jaz. 'Did he go to medical school here, at this university?'

'Yes and yes. He worked in general practice for many years, but had to retire when his sight started to fail. He always wanted to write a book about the history of medicine, but he never got round to it. I think he got a bit distracted searching for all these objects, to be honest – Good Lord!'

Mr Huxley was staring at the metal spiral.

'So *that's* where it got to,' he exclaimed. 'Now I don't feel such a duffer!' He turned to them. 'My little nephew broke his pogo stick and brought the bits in for me to fix while I was trying to pack these objects up. He *claimed* he'd gathered up all the broken pieces, but I couldn't for the life of me see how they all fitted together. That spring must have fallen into the carton – Oh, hello! You're Jaz's father? You must be so proud of your daughter! And I'm very pleased to meet *you*, Dr Radford –'

Rosy grabbed Jaz's sleeve and they dashed out of the room and down the stairs to the courtyard, where they were free to fall into fits of laughter.

'A pogo stick!' gasped Rosy, when she was able to talk again.

'We'd *never* have guessed that,' said Jaz. 'Not in a million years! Do you think we should take it out of the cabinet?'

'No way! Unless that kid wants it back. Anyway, it's related to medicine, isn't it? Exercising your leg muscles –'

'Getting out in the sunlight for a dose of vitamin D –'

'Exactly. Hey, let's go back and get some food. I was too nervous to eat anything before. We'll have to sneak in, though, because if Mr Huxley sees us and says anything else about that spiral, I'm going to start laughing again.'

They crept back up the stairs and peeked round the doorway. Ferdinand, Emmy and the electrician had gone home, but the others seemed to have settled in and were getting along famously. Lynette and the flying fox lady were discussing labrador training with Mr Huxley, while Rosy's mum and Dr Hudson stood nearby telling Mohammad all about medical scholarships. Dr Bennet, Maurice and Dr Adam were having a heated argument about the last Rugby World Cup, while over in the corner was Marcus and –

'Naomi!' whispered Rosy. 'Look, he's *flirting* with her! Should we go over and warn her off him?'

'Why? She doesn't seem to mind,' said Jaz. 'Anyway, I think he's nice. And quite handsome, really.'

'Handsome! Marcus?' Rosy scrutinised him. 'Yeah, he's not too bad,' she conceded, 'if you ignore the ridiculous T-shirts.'

But it was only as the girls were sneaking back out with the bowl of chips, a handful of chocolate-chip cookies and two glasses of cordial that they overheard the conversation that really made their day.

'No problem,' Mr Singh was saying to Ms Boydell. 'There aren't any dead trees to deal with, so it shouldn't take as long as the front garden. I'll type up a formal quote as soon as I get home and email it to you.'

Chapter Nineteen

'Excellent,' said Ms Boydell. 'I can't *wait* to be able to park my car round the back without all the paint getting scratched off the doors. Oh, and I meant to tell you, the Warden of St Peter's College was over here this morning, admiring the work we've had done out the front. I gave him your phone number.'

Laden as they were with snacks, Rosy and Jaz were unable to jump up and down and offer each other high fives, but their eyebrows said it all. They returned to the courtyard and settled happily on the edge of the pond, where the turtle – the one who'd started this whole thing off – crawled out of the water to stare at them.

'Malevolent,' Rosy called him, although Jaz maintained it hadn't really been his fault. And it had all worked out okay in the end, they agreed.

'Hey, is your dad working here tomorrow?' Rosy asked. 'Do you want to come with Mum and me to the markets? We wouldn't be leaving till about eleven.'

'No, he's finished everything he had to do out the front. But if they approve his quote, I guess he'll be here next week to start work around the back.'

'Oh, but I'm leaving on Monday!' said Rosy. Somehow she'd forgotten this in all the excitement. 'Dad and Gabrielle are picking me up on their way back home. Well, maybe you'll get to meet them, if your dad's coming in on Monday.'

'And I can meet your brother, too.'

'Yeah, he is pretty cute. I have missed him a bit, even if he is a giant pest sometimes. And I *really* missed

Dad. Ha, wait till I show him Dr Huxley's collection! He's going to love the Vesalius illustration. And you know, it was really my dad who helped us figure out that phrenological – Oh, here's *your* dad. You don't have to go already, do you? It's not even five o'clock.'

Mr Singh approached, tucking his mobile phone back in his pocket and looking troubled.

'Sorry, Jaz,' he said. 'We need to leave.'

'Right now?' said Jaz. 'But –'

'The nursing home called. She's had another fall. I'm just going to finish loading the truck – five minutes, okay?'

'Oh, Jaz,' cried Rosy, as Mr Singh strode off. 'I'm so sorry! Is it your grandma?'

Jaz shook her head, her eyes fixed on the flagstones. 'It's my mum,' she said.

Rosy blinked, then flung her arms around Jaz. After a moment, Jaz unfroze and hugged her back.

'That must be so hard for you,' Rosy said into Jaz's shoulder. She pulled back and stood up. 'But you don't have to tell me anything if you don't want to. Come on, let's get your bag from the flat.'

'No, I do want to tell you,' said Jaz. She took a deep breath. 'She has Huntington's disease.'

'Oh, that's *awful*,' said Rosy, even though she'd never heard of Huntington's disease. But it had to be awful, surely, if Jaz's mum needed special care? 'Does she live at the nursing home all the time, or only when she's feeling really bad, or …?' Rosy tugged Jaz towards the foyer, thinking it might be easier to talk if they were in motion.

Chapter Nineteen

'She moved there a year ago,' said Jaz, allowing herself to be led along. 'It's much better for her there. We couldn't look after her properly at home. She kept falling and hurting herself. And they have all sorts of specialist health people at the home who know what to do to help her.'

'Physiotherapists,' said Rosy, nodding, as she steered Jaz down the corridor.

'Yes, and occupational therapists and a speech pathologist. And most of the nurses are really nice. It's just ... you know. Sometimes I want to show her something I've done at school, but I have to wait till our next visit to tell her. And then when we get there, sometimes she's too tired to concentrate on what I'm saying –'

They'd reached Alison's flat, where Jaz grabbed her bag and glanced around for anything else she might have forgotten. 'Oh!' she exclaimed. 'My library books are still in your room!'

'Don't worry about that,' said Rosy, ushering her outside. 'I'll pack them all up and leave them in the office for your dad to collect next week. I'll even sort them according to their Dewey decimal numbers, okay? Look, your dad's waiting.'

He'd already started the engine and now leaned over to push open the passenger door of the ute.

'I might not get to see you on Monday,' said Jaz, biting her lip. 'They might have taken Mum to hospital.'

'Where's your pen? Look, here's my email,' said Rosy, writing it down. 'And give me yours. Then I can email you all my maths homework once term starts.'

'I'm not doing your homework for you!' said Jaz, almost laughing as she scribbled down her contact details.

'Jaz!' called her father.

'Coming!' she shouted back. She gave Rosy a quick, fierce hug, then ran off. Rosy stood there, waving, as the ute backed rapidly out of the car park.

'Bye!' cried Rosy. 'I hope your mum's okay! Let me know!'

But they had vanished in a cloud of dust. Rosy turned to see Alison walking towards her.

'Jaz's mum has Huntington's disease,' Rosy announced loudly. 'And ... and I don't even know what that *means*!'

Then she burst into tears.

CHAPTER TWENTY

'Did science promise happiness? I don't think so. It promised truth, and the question is whether the truth will ever make us happy.'
~ Émile Zola

Even when Rosy's mum had still been living with them, Rosy tended to go straight to her dad whenever she was hurt. Whether she'd gouged a hole in her leg with a screwdriver while trying to open a tin of paint or had just discovered her guinea pig squashed flat on the driveway, her dad usually knew how to make her feel better. Her mum, on the other hand, was inclined to ask awkward questions about where Rosy had got the screwdriver from and whether Rosy had shut the door of the guinea pig cage properly that morning. Alison was also uncomfortable with tears, possibly because she never cried herself. As Rosy had grown older, she'd decided that all of this was because her mother was a scientist and therefore not very good at emotions.

But the past two weeks had shown Rosy that scientists could be just as passionate and imaginative and expressive as artists were, so maybe Alison was simply a bit weird. Anyway, as Rosy's dad wasn't around to deal with this current crisis, Rosy had to make do with her mother patting her on the back rather clumsily and offering her a tissue. Then they went back inside and Rosy splashed cold water on her face and Alison made her some chocolate milk, which did result in her feeling slightly better. And, of course, Alison was also able to answer Rosy's many questions about Huntington's disease.

'It affects the part of the brain that controls how muscles work,' Alison explained. 'People with Huntington's disease have jerky, uncoordinated movements –'

'Oh, *chorea*,' said Rosy, remembering St Vitus's Dance.

'Yes, and their muscles can also get stuck in one position. And it's a degenerative disease, which means it gradually gets worse. It becomes hard for the person to walk around, or sit up straight, or sleep comfortably. It affects their ability to eat, to talk, even to breathe. There's medicine to treat some of the symptoms, but there's no cure. I think the most difficult part for families must be that it changes how the person thinks and behaves. People with Huntington's disease have problems remembering things, getting organised, coping with new situations. They can be impulsive and irritable and get very depressed –'

'Well, of *course* they do,' said Rosy. 'I'd be depressed, too, if I had to live in a nursing home and couldn't get out of bed or talk to people! But what causes it? Is it a virus?'

'No, no, it's genetic,' said Alison. 'Some people have a particular gene that's longer than normal. It

Chapter Twenty

tells their body to make a mutant protein that damages brain cells and that causes all the symptoms.'

'Genetic!' said Rosy with fresh horror. 'You mean ... it runs in families? But what about Jaz? Half of her genes come from her mum! Does that mean she has a fifty per cent chance of having that gene?'

'Well ... yes,' said Alison, looking very uncomfortable.

'Can she find out for sure? Does she already *know*?'

'There is a genetic test for Huntington's disease, but doctors don't usually test anyone younger than eighteen. Unless the child's already showing symptoms of the disease – which, of course, Jaz isn't.'

'But I think she'd want to find out anyway,' said Rosy. 'I *know* she would. She's really smart, she'd understand the results –'

'It's not that she wouldn't understand, Rosy. It's that it's such a huge decision to make, figuring out whether you want to be tested or not. Even adults need to attend months of counselling before they're allowed to have the test. It would change how Jaz thought about her whole life – careers, relationships, having children. Her family might start treating her differently, wrapping her up in cotton wool as though she were already sick. She could face discrimination from future employers or insurance companies ... If she finds out she carries the faulty gene, she can never un-know that fact.'

'But she might not have it.' Rosy clasped her hands together. 'There's an equal chance she doesn't. And then it would be an enormous *relief*. And she could get on with becoming a medical researcher and winning the Nobel Prize.'

'That's true,' said Alison. 'And even if she *did* have the faulty gene, she might not develop any symptoms till she was in her fifties or even older. And by then, there could be a cure.'

'But hang on,' Rosy said slowly, 'when did they discover Huntington's disease?'

'Oh, they've known there was such a thing as "hereditary chorea" for centuries. But they only identified the gene that caused it in 1993.'

'What?' said Rosy, getting mad all over again. 'Jaz was born years after that! If they'd already discovered the gene and knew that children had a fifty per cent chance of inheriting it, then why did Mr and Mrs Singh decide to have children at *all*?'

'Because they didn't *know*,' said Alison patiently. 'Jaz's mother didn't start to show any symptoms until she was thirty, and even then it took a year or two for doctors to work out it was Huntington's disease because there are lots of diseases that have similar symptoms. Jaz was already in preschool by then. There wasn't any clear history of the disease in the family. Jaz's grandfather on her mother's side died in a car accident in his fifties and now they think he was probably showing some signs of Huntington's disease before that, but no one had diagnosed it at the time.'

Rosy continued to glare. 'It's still horrible. It's just not *fair*.'

Chapter Twenty

'I know,' said Alison, with a sigh. 'Life isn't, a lot of the time. By the way, you have chocolate all over your mouth.' She handed Rosy another tissue.

Rosy scrubbed at her face, then flung the tissue at the bin. 'But why didn't Jaz *tell* me?' she burst out. 'All that time and she never said anything!'

'She *did* tell you, in the end,' said Alison. 'And her father said she never usually mentions it to anyone outside the family. Which makes it difficult for her at school, of course – imagine trying to get on with your studies and making friends when you're hiding such a big, important part of your life. He'd been really worried about her this past year, which is one of the reasons he didn't want to leave her at home by herself these holidays. But he said he hadn't seen her so happy and engrossed in anything for years, thanks to that project of yours. He could hear you two giggling up in your room all day. He told me how grateful he was that you were here.'

'He said that about *me*?' said Rosy. 'Really?'

'Things do tend to liven up when you're around,' said her mother dryly.

'Well, that's because I'm an artist,' said Rosy. 'I *am* very creative and imaginative …'

And then she had another one of her brilliant ideas.

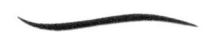

Rosy awoke the following morning to a startling flash of lightning, followed by the grumble of thunder. A steady pattering had started up on the roof and when she pushed open her window, she saw water streaming from the gargoyle's open mouth. By the time she and her mum had finished breakfast, rain was gushing down the windowpanes, washing away months of dust. Alison said they'd have to cancel their trip to the markets, but that was okay, because Rosy had other plans.

She lugged Alison's printer and a fresh ream of paper up to her room, then carefully packed up all of Jaz's library books and set them by the door. Then she turned on Methuselah and began printing out some of her very best photos – not just of Dr Huxley's thirteen objects, but also ones she'd taken on their travels around the university. There was Mephistopheles spitting into his pool and William Harvey's head outside the New Medical School and Gilgamesh trying to become immortal and ROENTGEN carved into the School of Physics and the patched-up lion and unicorn on the archway near the Nicholson Museum. She ran downstairs to the foyer to take a snapshot of Dr Huxley's swimming team photograph and then, tucked under an umbrella, dashed out to the courtyard to the turtle pond, where she coaxed the turtle into posing with a fresh lettuce leaf.

After that, Rosy went through all the bits and pieces that hadn't made it into their official notes on the Huxley Bequest. She printed out her screenplay about Professor Pasteur and Monsieur Beaker. She typed up a proper scientific report about her Midnight Visitor experiment. Then she went online to find photos of Vincent van Gogh's *The Starry Night* and Rembrandt's *The Anatomy Lesson of Dr Nicolaes Tulp* and Michelangelo's *Creation of Adam*, and she printed those out, too.

After a hasty lunch, she began pasting everything onto pieces of paper, adding labels in her very best handwriting. She left lots of blank spaces so she could add her own illustrations – a mummy stalking towards her desk with its arms stretched out, a vampire in a toga, James Lind as a zombie, Ned Kelly with his phrenological bumps showing through his helmet, Emily Rosa hoisting a trophy engraved with 'SKEPTIC OF THE YEAR', Alexander Fleming sneezing over his microscope so he could examine his own snot.

She drew Marcus in a lab coat, looking like the Future of Pharmacy, and Dr Bennet searching for her spectacles, even though they were on top of her head, and Sherlock Holmes with Watson (labelled, respectively, 'Rosy' and 'Jaz'). She drew a jar of marmalade labelled 'WARNING: CONTAINS GRAPEFRUIT!' and a jar of manuka honey sending out a flash of lightning to kill some evil yellow superbugs. She also tried to draw a possum sitting on her desk, but it turned out looking more like a cat, so she gave it flying goggles and a parachute. Then she gathered up her last few souvenirs – the tiny original scrap of Dr Huxley's notes that Rosy had snatched from the jaws of the turtle, Lynette's recipe for chocolate-chip cookies, a gum leaf from the possum's tree – and she stuck them in, as well.

It took her all of Saturday and quite a lot of Sunday, but finally she had a thick stack of papers, the edges of which she'd carefully punched holes in, then bound together with multicoloured twine. On the first page, she wrote,

For Jaz,
To remind you of the awesome time we had this summer!
From your good friend,
Rosalind Radford Smith

She looked at this for a moment, then added,

P. S. You are the Future of Science!!!

Then she remembered that even brilliant Nobel-Prize-winning scientists needed brilliant artistic people with exhausting vocabularies to communicate their ideas, so she changed the last 'You' to 'We'. And then she put her book on top of Jaz's library collection, ready to be carried down to the office, first thing on Monday.

AUTHOR'S NOTE

'Science will go on whether we are pessimistic, or are optimistic, as I am. I know that great, interesting and valuable discoveries can be made and will be made ... and I am awaiting them, full of curiosity and enthusiasm.'
~ Linus Pauling

Rosy, Jaz and all the people working at the university are figments of my imagination, but the historical people, medical discoveries and scientific facts described in this book are all real and the university bears a strong resemblance to the University of Sydney. If you walk around the University of Sydney's Camperdown campus, you too will be able to see Mephistopheles spitting in his pool, Gilgamesh strangling his lion, William Harvey and Louis Pasteur (or at least, their stone heads) sitting outside the Blackburn Building, the mummy of the boy Horus in the Nicholson Museum, the Future of Pharmacy picture in the Pharmacy building and exhibitions of rare books in Fisher Library.

Unfortunately, you won't be able to look at Louis Pasteur's flask of broth because it's in the Pathology Museum, which isn't open to the public – although the curator kindly allowed me to view the collection when I was writing this book. The Macleay Museum was closed down in 2016, in preparation for a move to a big new university museum, due to open in 2019. Hopefully, the stuffed possum, pickled rats and giant tapeworm will be displayed in a prominent position. There is no such place as New College, but people who know the University of Sydney may be able to guess which residential college it is based upon (and yes, the real college does have a turtle pond).

This book is a brief history of how medicine moved from superstition to science. It is not the whole story of medicine, health or science. It's full of my own personal interests and biases, and I'm sure some of it will be out of date by the time you read this, because new medical discoveries are being made every day. *Dr Huxley's Bequest* is simply a starting point for your own investigations into this fascinating subject.

I've included a bibliography so you can see where I found all of my information. Some of the articles from scientific journals can be a bit difficult to understand unless you have a science degree, but most of the books and newspaper articles that I've listed are fairly reader-friendly. If you're interested in reading more, I recommend starting with *Bad science* by Ben Goldacre, then trying *Taking the medicine* by Druin Burch, *Killer germs* by Barry and David Zimmerman and *Trick or treatment* by Simon Singh and Edzard Ernst.

Finally, I'd like to thank everyone who helped me put this book together, especially Helena Newton for her invaluable editorial assistance, Nada Backovic for her cover design expertise, Diana Murray for interior design help and The Arts Law Centre of Australia for legal advice.

BIBLIOGRAPHY

Alvarez, Luis W. (1987). *Alvarez: Adventures of a physicist*. New York, NY: Basic Books.

Ashburton Thompson, J. (1901). A contribution to the aetiology of plague. *The Journal of Hygiene*, 1(2), 153–167.

Atwood, K. C. (2004). Bacteria, ulcers, and ostracism? *H. pylori* and the making of a myth. *Skeptical Inquirer*, 28(6). Retrieved from http://www.csicop.org/si/show/bacteria_ulcers_and_ostracism_h._pylori_and_the_making_of_a_myth/

Austin, J. J., Ross, A. J., Smith, A. B., Fortey, R. A. & Thomas, R. H. (1997). Problems of reproducibility – does geologically ancient DNA survive in amber-preserved insects? *Proceedings of the Royal Society B: Biological Sciences*, 264(1381), 467–474.

Australian Government Department of Health. (2013). *The Australian immunisation handbook* (10th ed.). Retrieved from http://www.immunise.health.gov.au/internet/immunise/publishing.nsf/Content/Handbook10-home

Australian Huntington's Disease Youth Alliance. (2012). *Our HD space*. Retrieved from http://www.ourhdspace.org/

Bailey, D. G., Dresser, G. & Arnold, J. M. O. (2012). Grapefruit-medication interactions: Forbidden fruit or avoidable consequences? *Canadian Medical Association Journal*, 185(4), 309–316. Retrieved from http://www.cmaj.ca/content/185/4/309.full

The British Museum. (no date). Faience wedjat eye. Retrieved from http://culturalinstitute.britishmuseum.org/asset-viewer/faience-wedjat-eye/PQHDiqnrxByGgA?hl=en

Brody, J. E. (2012, August 20). Medical radiation soars, with risks often overlooked. *The New York Times*. Retrieved from http://well.blogs.nytimes.com/2012/08/20/medical-radiation-soars-with-risks-often-overlooked/

Bronzetti, G., Canzi, A. & Picchio, F. M. (2002). Van Gogh, Doctor Gachet, and digitalis: A self-diagnostic portrait? *Cardiovascular Drug Reviews*, 20(3), 233–236.

Brown, K. (2005). *Penicillin Man: Alexander Fleming and the antibiotic revolution*. Stroud, UK: Sutton Publishing.

Bruce-Chwatt, L. J. (1981). Alphonse Laveran's discovery 100 years ago and today's global fight against malaria. *Journal of the Royal Society of Medicine*, 74(7), 531–536.

Burch, D. (2009). *Taking the medicine: A short history of medicine's beautiful idea and our difficulty swallowing it*. London: Vintage Books.

Burns, L. (2007). Gunther von Hagens' BODY WORLDS: Selling beautiful education. *The American Journal of Bioethics*, 7(4), 12–23.

Clarke, P. (2008). Aboriginal healing practices and Australian bush medicine. *Journal of the Anthropological Society of South Australia*, 33, 3–38.

Corderoy, A. (2013, March 9–10). Anti-vaccination physicians training chiropractors. *The Sydney Morning Herald*. p. 9.

Davies, J. (2013, December 28–29). Rise of the superbugs. *The Sydney Morning Herald*. p. 5.

Dawkins, R. (2006). *The God delusion*. London: Bantam Press.

Desmond, A. (1997). *Huxley: Evolution's high priest*. London: Michael Joseph.

Doherty, B. (2012, December 21–23). Children the losers in deadly stand-off. *The Sydney Morning Herald*. p. 10.

Ehrenreich, B. & English, D. (1972). *Witches, midwives and nurses: A history of women healers*. New York, NY: The Feminist Press.

Einstein, A. (1952). Letter to Carl Seelig, March 11, 1952, Einstein Archives 39–013. Cited in Isaacson, W. (2008). *Einstein: His life and universe*. New York, NY: Simon and Schuster.

Elion, G. B. (1993). Quoted in McGrayne, S. B. (1998). *Nobel Prize women in science: Their lives, struggles, and momentous discoveries*: Second edition. Washington, DC: The National Academies Press.

Evans, I., Thornton, H. & Chalmers, I. (2010). *Testing treatments: Better research for better healthcare*. London: Pinter & Martin.

Flanagan, S. (1995). Hildegard von Bingen (1098–1179). In J. Harden & W. Hasty (Eds.). *Dictionary of literary bibliography*, Vol. 148: German writers and works of the early middle ages, 800–1170 (pp. 59–73). Detroit, MI: Gale Research.

Garrison, D., Hast, M. & Northwestern University. (2003). *On the fabric of the human body: An annotated translation of the 1543 and 1555 editions of Andreas Vesalius' De Humani Corporis Fabrica*. Retrieved from http://vesalius.northwestern.edu/index.html

Goldacre, B. (2007). Benefits and risks of homoeopathy. *The Lancet*, 370, 1672–1673.

Goldacre, B. (2009). *Bad science*. London: Fourth Estate.

Gordon, H. L. (1897). *Sir James Young Simpson and chloroform (1811–1870)*. London: T. Fisher Unwin.

Haddad, S. I. & Khairallah, A. A. (1936). A forgotten chapter in the history of the circulation of the blood. *Annals of Surgery*, 104(1), 1–8.

Haliova, B. & Ziskind, B. (2005). *Medicine in the days of the pharaohs*. Cambridge, MA: The Belknap Press of Harvard University.

Hamlet, W. (1914). Letter written by the New South Wales Government Analyst, on behalf of the New South Wales Department of Public Health, November 18, 1914. Held in the collection of the Interactive Centre for Human Diseases (Pathology Museum), The University of Sydney.

Hogarth, M., Lagan, B. & O'Neill, J. (1988, November 22). Dr William McBride, the man and the myths: McBride projects failed to win govt funds. *The Sydney Morning Herald*, p. 12.

Jeffreys, D. (2004). *Aspirin: The story of a wonder drug*. London: Bloomsbury.

Jeffries, S. (2002, March 19). The naked and the dead. *The Guardian*. Retrieved from http://www.theguardian.com/education/2002/mar/19/arts.highereducation

Lévi-Strauss, C. (1990). *The raw and the cooked: Mythologiques*, Volume One. Translated by John and Doreen Weightman. Chicago, IL: University of Chicago Press.

Lind, J. (1753). *A treatise of the scurvy: in three parts: containing an inquiry into the nature, causes and cure, of that disease: together with a critical and chronological view of what has been published on the subject*. Edinburgh: Printed by Sands, Murray and Cochran for A. Kincaid and A. Donaldson.

Link, K. (2005). *The vaccine controversy: The history, use, and safety of vaccinations*. Westport, Conn: Praeger.

Lorenz, K. (1966). *On aggression*. Translated by Marjorie Kerr Wilson. New York, NY: Harcourt, Brace, and World.

Maddox, B. (2003). *Rosalind Franklin: The dark lady of DNA*. New York, NY: HarperCollins.

Manheimer, E., Wieland, S., Kimbrough, E., Chang, K. & Berman, B. M. (2009). Evidence from the Cochrane Collaboration for Traditional Chinese Medicine

Therapies. *Journal of Alternative and Complementary Medicine*, 15(9), 1001–1014.

McKenzie, N. & Baker, R. (2012, July 26). The 50-year global cover-up. *The Sydney Morning Herald*. Retrieved from http://www.smh.com.au/national/the-50year-global-coverup-20120725-22r5c.html

Medical Tribunal of New South Wales. (1996). *A decision of the Medical Tribunal of NSW in relation to: Dr William McBride and The Medical Practice Act* (April 29, 1996). Retrieved from www.mcnsw.org.au/resources/378/McBride.pdf

Minakawa, N., Dida, G. O., Sonye, G. O., Futami, K. and Kaneko, S. (2008) Unforeseen misuses of bed nets in fishing villages along Lake Victoria. *Malaria Journal*, 7(165). Retrieved from http://www.malariajournal.com/content/7/1/165

Minkowski, W. L. (1992). Women healers of the Middle Ages: Selected aspects of their history. *American Journal of Public Health*, 82(2), 288–295.

Mozley, A. (1966). Huxley, Thomas Henry (1825–1895). In National Centre of Biography (Ed.) *Australian Dictionary of Biography*. Canberra: Australian National University. Retrieved from http://adb.anu.edu.au/biography/huxley-thomas-henry-2219/text2883

Nájera, J. A., González-Silva, M. & Alonso, P. L. (2011). Some lessons for the future from the Global Malaria Eradication Programme (1955–1969). *Public Library of Science Medicine* 8(1), e1000412. Retrieved from http://www.plosmedicine.

org/article/info%3Adoi%2F10.1371%2Fjournal.pmed.1000412

Ndi, C. P., Semple, S. J., Griesser, H. J. & Barton, M. D. (2007). Antimicrobial activity of some Australian plant species from the genus Eremophila. *Journal of Basic Microbiology*, 47, 158–164.

O'Shaughnessy, P. T. (2008). Parachuting cats and crushed eggs: The controversy over the use of DDT to control malaria. *American Journal of Public Health*, 98(11), 1940–1948.

Palombo, E. A. & Semple, S. J. (2001). Antibacterial activity of traditional Australian medicinal plants. *Journal of Ethnopharmacology*, 77:2–3, 151–157.

Park, R. H. R. & Park, M. P. (1990). Saint Vitus' dance: vital misconceptions by Sydenham and Bruegel. *Journal of the Royal Society of Medicine*, 83, 512–515.

Pauling, L. (1947). Lecture at Yale University, 'Chemical Achievement and Hope for the Future'. Published in Baitsell, G. A. (Ed.). (1949). *Science in Progress*: Sixth Series. New Haven, Conn: Yale University Press.

Pollak, J. (2006, September–October). A short essay in defence of the imagination. *EMU Newsletter*. Retrieved from http://www.jenny-pollak.com/news-galleries/

Pollard, J. (Ed.). (2000). *A caregiver's handbook for advanced-stage Huntington's disease*. Cambridge, Canada: Huntington Society of Canada.

Porter, R. (1997). *The greatest benefit to mankind: A medical history of humanity from antiquity to the present*. London: HarperCollins.

Quave, C. L., Plano, L. R. W., Pantuso, T. & Bennett, B. C. (2008). Effects of extracts from Italian medicinal plants on planktonic growth, biofilm formation and adherence of methicillin-resistant *Staphylococcus aureus*. *Journal of Ethnopharmacology*, 118(3), 418–428.

Raoult, D., Aboudharam, G., Crubézy, E., Larrouy, G., Ludes, B. & Drancourt, M. (2000). Molecular identification by 'suicide PCR' of *Yersinia pestis* as the agent of Medieval Black Death. *Proceedings of the National Academy of Sciences*, 97(23), 12800–12803.

Rosa, L., Rosa, E., Sarner, L. & Barrett, S. (1998). A close look at Therapeutic Touch. *Journal of the American Medical Association*, 279(13), 1005–1010.

Sagan, C. (1990). Why we need to understand science. *Skeptical Inquirer*, 14(3). Retrieved from http://www.csicop.org/si/show/why_we_need_to_understand_science

Samarasekera, U. (2007). Pressure grows against homoeopathy in the UK. *The Lancet*, 370, 1677–1678.

Science Museum, London. (no date). Dried smallpox vaccine, England, 1979. Retrieved from http://www.sciencemuseum.org.uk/broughttolife/objects/display.aspx?id=6003

Shah, S. (2010). *Fever: How malaria has ruled humankind for 500,000 years*. Sydney: Allen & Unwin.

Shahid, S., Bleam, R., Bessarab, D. & Thompson, S.C. (2010). 'If you don't believe it, it won't help you': use of bush medicine in treating cancer among Aboriginal people in Western Australia. *Journal of Ethnobiology and Ethnomedicine*, 6:18. Retrieved from http://www.ethnobiomed.com/content/6/1/18

Shapiro, R. (2008). *Suckers: How alternative medicine makes fools of us all*. London: Harvill Secker.

Singh, S. & Ernst, E. (2008). *Trick or treatment: The undeniable facts about alternative medicine*. New York, NY: W. W. Norton & Co.

Smith, D. (2011, January 8–9). Exploring the genetic jungle can be fraught with danger. *The Sydney Morning Herald*, pp. 6–7.

Smith, T. C. (2008, January 16–19). Did *Yersinia pestis* really cause Black Plague? Retrieved from http://scienceblogs.com/aetiology/2008/01/16/did_yersinia_pestis_really_cau/

Somerville, J. M. (2005). Dr Sophia Jex-Blake and the Edinburgh School of Medicine for Women, 1886–1898. *Journal of the Royal College of Physicians of Edinburgh*, 35, 261–267.

Stille, D. R. (1997). *Extraordinary women of medicine*. New York, NY: Children's Press, Grolier Publishing.

Suk, I. & Tamargo, R. (2010). Concealed neuroanatomy in Michelangelo's Separation of Light From Darkness in the Sistine Chapel. *Neurosurgery*, 66(5), 851–861.

Szasz, T. S. (1973). *The second sin*. New York, NY: Anchor Press, Doubleday.

Tanner, S. T. (2011). *100 Van Gogh masterpieces*. London: Flame Tree Publishing.

Tröhler, U. (2003). James Lind and scurvy: 1747 to 1795. *James Lind Library Bulletin: Commentaries on the history of treatment evaluation*. Retrieved from www.jameslindlibrary.org

University of Sydney. (2014). Reading heads and ruling passions: An exhibition on phrenology. Retrieved from http://sydney.edu.au/museums/exhibitions-events/phrenology.shtml

University of Sydney. (2014). Faculty of Medicine Online Museum and Archive. Retrieved from http://sydney.edu.au/medicine/museum/mwmuseum/index.php

Usher, S. M. & Chieveley-Williams, S. (2004). 'A Yankee dodge': the first British public demonstration of anaesthesia. *Grand Rounds*, 4, 12–14.

Van der Weyden, M. B., Armstrong, R. M. & Gregory, A. T. (2005). The 2005 Nobel Prize in Physiology or Medicine. *Medical Journal of Australia*, 183(11/12). Retrieved from www.mja.com.au/journal/2005/183/11/2005-nobel-prize-physiology-or-medicine

Wickenden, J. V. S. (2011). The strange disappearances of James Lind. *James Lind Library Bulletin: Commentaries on the history of treatment evaluation*. Retrieved from www.jameslindlibrary.org

Wilson, D. (2002). Explaining the 'Criminal': Ned Kelly's death mask. *The La Trobe Journal*, 69, 51–58.

Zimmerman, B. E. & Zimmerman, D. J. (2003). *Killer germs: Microbes and diseases that threaten humanity*. New York, NY: McGraw Hill.

Zola, É. (1893). Address at the Students' Association Banquet, May 18, 1893. Cited in Jacob, F. (1998). *Of flies, mice and men*. Translated by Giselle Weiss. Cambridge, Mass: Harvard University Press.

INDEX

A

A Treatise of the Scurvy by James Lind, 24, 163–167, 172–175

acupuncture, 225–226

AIDS. *See* HIV/AIDS

alchemy, 86–89, 124

allergies, 194, 200, 249, 288

al-Razi, Muhammad ibn Zakariya (Rhazes), 89

al-Tabari, 'Ali ibn Rabban, 89

alternative therapies. *See* chiropractic, homeopathy, reiki, Therapeutic Touch

Alvarez, Luis, 13

An Account of the Foxglove and Some of its Medical Uses by William Withering, 220

anaesthetics, 150, 153–156

anatomy, history of, 52–53, 55–57, 91–104

ancient Egypt, medicine, 35–39, 48, 55, 153, 210, 265

ancient Greece, medicine, 37, 47, 48–53, 72, 81, 89, 171, 223, 235

ancient India, medicine, 49, 55, 153

ancient Rome, medicine, 37, 54–57, 68, 87, 95, 153, 265

ancient Sumer, medicine, 153

Andry, Nicholas, 132

animals, use in medicine, 38, 52–54, 55, 57, 72, 80, 81–82, 95, 110, 136–140, 154, 178, 191–192, 214, 216, 226–227, 233, 238–239, 273–274, 291

Anson, George, 167

anthrax, 133, 139, 140, 142

antibiotics, 148, 149, 153, 231–239, 291–292

antisepsis, 150, 157–161

apothecary, 89, 211, 223

Arabic medicine. *See* Islam, role in medicine

Aristotle, 52–53, 55, 72

Armstrong, William, 75

artemisinin, 227, 271

arteries. *See* blood circulation system

Asclepius (god), 50

Ashburton Thompson, John, 75

aspirin, 38, 199, 209–213, 219

Aspro. *See* aspirin

asthma, 200, 220, 249

astrology, 81, 88

Australian Aboriginal traditional medicine, 219, 239

autism, 247–249, 251

Avicenna (Abu 'Ali al-Husayn ibn 'Abd Allah ibn Sina), 87–89

Ayurvedic medicine, 49

B

bacteria, 71, 130, 132–139, 142–145, 147, 149, 159, 161, 181, 232–239, 291–292. *See also* cholera, diphtheria, *E. Coli*, *Helicobacter pylori*, leprosy, MRSA, plague, pneumonia, puerperal fever, *Staphylococcus aureus*, tetanus, tuberculosis, typhoid, *Yersinia pestis*

Bayer, 211–214

Becquerel, Henri, 281

Bionic Ear (cochlear implant), 295

birth control pills. *See* contraception

Black Death, 70–75, 81. *See also* plague

Blackburn, Elizabeth, 290

Blane, Gilbert, 175

blood circulation system, 52–53, 57, 95, 108–115, 158, 169, 201, 213, 219, 266, 270, 286

bloodletting, 56–57, 70, 72, 73, 80, 109, 197, 200, 225

Body Worlds. *See* von Hagens, Gunther

body-snatching, 99

Borgognoni, Theodoric, 157

Borna virus, 149

brain. *See* nervous system

British Museum, 36

Broca, Paul, 192

Brotzu, Giuseppe, 235

Bruegel the Elder, Pieter, 68–69

Burke, William, 99

C

cancer, 45–46, 101, 148, 149, 169, 179, 201, 205, 215, 282, 294

capillaries. *See* blood circulation system

Captain Moonlite, 190

carbon-dating, 39

Causae et Curae by Hildegard of Bingen, 81

Caventou, Joseph, 267

Celsus, 54, 87, 210

Chain, Ernst, 233–234

Chamberland, Charles, 139

Chemie Grünenthal, 214–215

chemotherapy, 294

China, traditional medicine, 223, 224–227, 271

chiropractic, 193, 200–201

Chirurgia by Theodoric Borgognoni, 157

chloroform, 155–156

chloroquine, 271

chocolate, as medicine, 219

cholera, 130, 131, 133, 137–139, 140, 142–143, 156, 197

chorea. *See* Huntington's disease, St Vitus's Dance

Christianity, role in medicine, 68–70, 71–72, 74, 76, 80–86, 95, 97–98

Index

chromosome. *See* DNA (deoxyribonucleic acid)

cigarettes. *See* smoking, effect on health

cinchona (Peruvian bark), 194, 210, 267

Clarke, William, 155

Colombo, Realdo, 115

contraception, 294

control group, 117, 173–174, 205, 214, 225, 247. *See also* scientific method

Cook, James, 176

Cordus, Valerius, 154

correlation and causation, 204–205, 251

cot death. *See* SIDS

cowpox, 138, 242–243

CPR (cardiopulmonary resuscitation), 294

Creation of Adam by Michelangelo, 97–98

Crick, Francis, 284, 290

CT (computed tomography) imaging, 34, 39, 282

Curie, Marie, 281

Curie, Pierre, 281

D

dancing mania, 68–70

Darwin, Charles, 120, 241

Darwin, Francis, 229

Davy, Humphry, 154

Dawkins, Richard, 257

DDT (dichlorodiphenyltrichloroethane) insecticide, 273–274

Debendox, 216

De Humani Corporis Fabrica by Andreas Vesalius, 91–97, 98–99, 102, 108–109, 171

De Materia Medica by Dioscorides, 171

De Motu Cordis (On the Motion of the Heart) by William Harvey, 108–115

dentistry and teeth, 34, 38, 39, 52, 71, 80, 154, 166–167, 282, 295

diabetes, 181, 249, 295

diet and nutrition, 39, 48–49, 55, 89, 135–136, 173–181, 238, 271, 286, 291

digitalis, 220–222

Dioscorides, Pedanius, 171, 210

diphtheria, 145, 252

dissection, 52–54, 55, 94–104

DNA (deoxyribonucleic acid), 263–264, 270, 280, 283–284, 286–287, 289, 290, 308–309

Domagk, Gerhard, 235

Down Syndrome, 287

drug resistance, 236–239, 271–272, 275

Dumas, Jean-Baptiste, 177–178

E

E. Coli (Escherichia Coli), 238

Ebers papyri, 37

Ebola, 148

Edwin Smith papyri, 37

Egypt. *See* ancient Egypt, medicine

Einstein, Albert, 31

Elion, Gertrude, 277

Emerson, Ralph Waldo, 219
epidemic, 69, 74, 75, 126, 143, 197, 244, 265
epilepsy, 54, 68–69, 83, 191, 220, 251
Epstein-Barr virus, 148
Erasistratus, 53
ergotism, 69–70
ether, 154–156

F

Fabricius ab Aquapendente, Hieronymus, 115
Faust, 2, 85–86
Felicie, Jacqueline, 83
Ferrier, David, 191–192
Fisher Library, University of Sydney, 167, 168, 171, 315
fleas, 71, 75, 265, 267
Fleming, Alexander, 232–234, 236, 300
Florey, Howard, 233–234
flu. *See* influenza
fluoride in water supply, 295
Forster, Thomas, 189
Fowler, Lorenzo, 189–190
Fowler, Orson, 189
foxglove. *See* digitalis
Fracastoro, Girolamo, 132
Franklin, Rosalind, 284–285, 290
Funk, Casimir, 178

G

G6PD deficiency diseases, 270–271
Gage, Phineas, 192–193

Galen of Pergamon, 54–57, 72, 87, 88, 95, 108–110, 157, 210, 223
Gall, Franz Joseph, 189
garlic, as medicine, 164, 174, 219
gastric ulcers, 169, 291–292
genes. *See* DNA, genetic testing
genetic testing, 286–287, 289–290, 309–310
germ theory, 132, 135–136, 159, 200
germs. *See* bacteria, protozoa, viruses
Gilgamesh, 124, 315
ginger, as medicine, 219, 220
Golgi, Camillo, 267–268
grapefruit, interactions with medicines, 220

H

haemophilia, 213
Hahnemann, Samuel, 194–195, 210
Hamilton. A. S., 190
Hamlet, William (Director General of Public Health), 130
Hare, William, 99
Harvey, William, 108–115, 315
Haydn, Joseph, 191
heart. *See* blood circulation system
Heatley, Norman, 233–234
Helicobacter pylori, 291–292
hepatitis, 148, 243
herd immunity, 249–250. *See also* immunisation
heroin, 213–214

Index

Herophilus, 53
Hesse, Fanny, 144
Hildegard of Bingen, 76, 81–82
Hippocrates, 47–51, 55, 88, 204, 210
Hippocratic oath, 47, 50
HIV/AIDS, 147, 148, 249, 293
homeopathy, 193–199, 203, 204, 206, 210
honey, use in medicine, 38, 49, 219, 238–239
Hopkins, Frederick Gowland, 178
Horus (god), 33–37
human papillomavirus (HPV), 148
humours, humoural theory, 49, 55–56, 81
Huntington's disease, 304–305, 308–310
Huxley, Thomas Henry, 61, 107, 120, 125, 182–183, 235, 279
Hygieia (goddess), 50
hypothesis, 43, 71, 116–119, 124, 148, 182, 202, 217, 247, 258–261, 289, 291–292, 296–297. *See also* scientific method

I

Ibn al-Nafis, 'Ala' al-Din, 114–115
Ibn Sina. *See* Avicenna
immunisation, 27, 138–141, 148, 200, 241–252, 273
inflammation, 54, 87, 157
influenza, 148, 237, 251
insulin, 295
Islam, role in medicine, 88–89, 114–115, 223

J

Jenner, Edward, 242–243
Jennings, Margaret, 233–234
Jex-Blake, Sophia, 279
Joliot-Curie, Irène, 281
Judaism, role in medicine, 72, 115

K

Kelly, Ned, 190
Kemp, Ursula, 84
Kircher, Athanasius, 132
Koch, Robert, 141–142, 144–145, 157

L

laudanum. *See* opium
Laveran, Alphonse, 267–268
leeches, 80
Leonardo da Vinci, 96–98
leprosy, 81, 83, 145, 215
Lévi-Strauss, Claude, 43
Lind, James, 167, 172–177
Lister, Joseph, 159, 235
Liston, Robert, 155
Long, Crawford, 155
Lorenz, Konrad, 289
Lunin, Nikolai Ivanovich, 178
Lusitano, Amato, 115
lysosomes, 232–233

M

Macleay Museum, University of Sydney, 125–126, 316
malaria, 39, 194, 209, 227, 265–275
Malleus Maleficarum by Institoris and Sprenger, 83, 171

manuka honey. *See* honey, use in medicine

Marshall, Barry, 290–292

McBride, William, 215–217, 296

measles, 148, 246–248, 252

medieval Europe, medicine, 68–74, 76, 80–84, 147, 153, 223

Meister, Joseph, 141

mental illness, 140, 149, 154, 159, 179, 220–221, 288, 308. *See also* schizophrenia

Mephistopheles, 2, 85–86, 315

mesmerism, 154

miasma theory, 142, 145, 159

Michelangelo Buonarroti, 97–98

microbiology. *See* bacteria, protozoa, viruses

microscopes, 114, 126, 132, 140, 144, 145, 161

Middle Ages. *See* medieval Europe, medicine

midwifery, 80, 83, 158

MMR (Measles Mumps Rubella) vaccine, 247–248, 251

Morton, William, 155

mosquitos, 264–268, 270, 272–275

Moyer, Andrew, 234

MRI (magnetic resonance imaging), 282

MRSA (Methicillin-resistant *Staphylococcus aureus*), 236–239

mummies (ancient Egyptian), 34–35, 36, 39, 315

mumps, 247–248, 251

N

nervous system, 52, 53, 97–98, 169, 186–187, 189–193, 201, 266, 282, 308–309

Nicholas, George, 212

Nicholson Museum, University of Sydney, 32–39, 82, 268, 278, 315

Nightingale, Florence, 159

nitrous oxide, 154

Nobel Prize, 178, 203, 234, 236, 268, 281, 284–285, 290–291

Nostradamus, 73

O

Ombredanne inhaler, 123, 149–150, 156. *See also* ether

Ombredanne, Louis, 156

opium, 38, 57, 88, 153

organ donation, organ transplants, 100–101, 288

Orr-Ewing, Jean, 233–234

P

Pagenstecher, Johann, 211

Paine, Cecil, 233

Palmer, Daniel David, 200

Panacea (god), 50

pandemic, 70–75, 148

Paracelsus, 87–88, 154, 209

Paré, Ambroise, 157–158, 172–173

Pasteur Institute, 130, 141, 147

Pasteur, Louis, 115, 129–141, 142, 144, 145, 150, 157, 159, 235, 315

pasteurisation, 115, 131, 133–136, 142

Pauling, Linus, 315

Pelletier, Pierre, 267

penicillin, 231–234, 236–237, 254

peppermint, as medicine, 219, 220

Petri dish, 145, 232

Petri, Julius, 145

pharmacy, history of, 209–227, 315. *See also* apothecary

phrenology, 188–191, 193

Physica by Hildegard of Bingen, 81

Physiognomical System by Johann Spurzheim, 189

placebos and placebo effect, 198–199, 225–226

plague, 70–76, 81, 126, 142, 145, 147, 265, 267, 274. *See also* Black Death

Plasmodia, 267, 270–275

pneumonia, 145

poliomyelitis, 148, 244–246, 252, 273

Pollak, Jenny, 91

Pouchet, Félix, 135

Prior, Matthew, 207

protozoa, 269–270. *See also* Plasmodia

puerperal fever (childbed fever), 158

Q

quarantine, 74

quinine, 267, 271

R

rabies, 139–141

radiotherapy, 282

randomisation, 173, 197, 205, 225, 247. *See also* scientific method

Rasputin, 213

rats, 71, 75–76, 126, 178, 274, 316

RBT (random breath testing) for drivers, effect on health, 295

reiki, 201

Rembrandt, 96–97

resistance of microbes to drugs. *See* drug resistance

Rhazes. *See* al-Razi, Muhammad ibn Zakariya

rickets, 178–179

Rod of Asclepius, 50, 108

Roentgen, Wilhelm, 278, 280–281

Rosa, Emily, 201–203

Ross, Ronald, 267–268

Roux, Pierre, 140

rubella, 247–248, 252

S

Sabin, Albert, 245

Sagan, Carl, 163

Salk, Jonas, 244

Schatz, Albert, 235

schizophrenia, 149, 288

scientific method, 39, 43, 52, 96, 108–112, 116–119, 124, 161, 163, 172–174, 182, 201–206, 214, 216–217, 225, 247, 258–261, 291–292. *See also* control group, hypothesis, randomisation, variables

scurvy, 163–167, 172–176

seatbelts in cars, effect on health, 295

Semmelweis, Ignaz, 158–159

Separation of Light from Darkness by Michelangelo, 98
Servetus, Michael, 115
Shen Nung, 223, 224
Shmith, Henry Woolf, 212
sickle-cell anaemia, 270
SIDS (Sudden Infant Death Syndrome), cot death, 294
Simpson, James Young, 155
smallpox, 39, 138, 148, 241–244, 245, 252
Smith, Edwin, papyri, 37
smoking, effect on health, 101, 168–169, 286, 288
Snow, John, 142–144, 156
Spurzheim, Johann, 189
St Anthony, 70
St Anthony's Fire. *See* ergotism
St Cosmas, 153
St Damian, 153
St Vitus, 67–69
St Vitus's Dance, 68–69, 308. *See also* dancing mania
Staphylococcus aureus, 236–239. *See also* MRSA
stomach ulcers. *See* gastric ulcers
Stone, Edward, 209–210
superbugs (drug-resistant bacteria), 236–239. *See also* MRSA
surgery, history of, 37, 47, 50, 54, 88, 89, 94, 120, 149–150, 152–161, 167, 172–173, 181, 198, 279
sweet wormwood, 227, 271
Sydenham's chorea. *See* St Vitus's Dance
Syme, James, 154
Szasz, Thomas, 77, 185
Szent-Györgyi, Albert, 178

T

tapeworms, 39, 126, 316
teeth. *See* dentistry
temperament, 55–56, 59. *See also* humours
Tennyson, Alfred, Lord, 151
tetanus, 145
thalidomide, 214–217
The Anatomy Lesson of Dr Nicolaes Tulp by Rembrandt, 96–97
The Epileptic Women of Molenbeek by Pieter Bruegel the Elder, 68–69
The Night Café by Vincent van Gogh, 221
The Starry Night by Vincent van Gogh, 221
The Yellow House by Vincent van Gogh, 221
Therapeutic Touch, 201–203
thiomersal, 249
Tidswell, Frank, 75
Titian, 96
Traditional Chinese Medicine (TCM). *See* China, traditional medicine
tuberculosis, 142
Twain, Mark, 190
typhoid, 145

U

ultrasound, 198, 282

V

vaccination. *See* immunisation

vaccinia, 243. *See also* smallpox, cowpox

van Calcar, Jan Stephan, 96

van Gogh, Vincent, 221–222

van Leeuwenhoek, Anton, 132

variables, 117, 173, 205, 258, 259. *See also* scientific method

Varro, 132

veins. *See* blood circulation system

Vesalius, Andreas, 91–99, 102, 108, 109

viruses, 140, 147–149, 237, 242–247, 249–250, 284, 308. *See also* Borna virus, cowpox, Ebola, Epstein-Barr virus, hepatitis, HIV/AIDS, human papillomavirus, influenza, measles, poliomyelitis, rabies, smallpox, vaccinia

vitamins, 166, 167, 175–181

von Bergmann, Ernst, 159–160

von Hagens, Gunther, 101–104

von Hohenheim, Theophrastus. *See* Paracelsus

W

Wakefield, Andrew, 247–248

Waksman, Zolman, 235

Walker, Mary Edwards (Civil War surgeon), 279

Warren, John, 155

Warren, Robin, 290–292

Watson, James, 284, 290

Wells, Horace, 154

Wernicke, Carl, 192

WHO. *See* World Health Organization

whooping cough, 250

willow, use in medicine, 38, 209–210

witches and witchcraft, 80, 83–86. *See also Malleus Maleficarum*

Withering, William, 220

women in medicine and science, history of, 76, 80–85, 223, 277, 279, 281, 284–285. *See also* Blackburn, Elizabeth; Curie, Marie; Elion, Gertrude; Felicie, Jacqueline; Franklin, Rosalind; Hesse, Fanny; Hildegard of Bingen; Jennings, Margaret; Jex-Blake, Sophia; Joliot-Curie, Irène; Kemp, Ursula; Nightingale, Florence; Orr-Ewing, Jean; Rosa, Emily; Walker, Mary Edwards

World Health Organization, 244, 245, 273–274

X

X-rays, 201, 281–282

Y

Yersinia pestis, 71

Z

Zika, 148

Zola, Émile, 307

ABOUT THE AUTHOR

Michelle Cooper is the author of *The Rage of Sheep* and *The Montmaray Journals* trilogy. The first Montmaray novel, *A Brief History of Montmaray*, won a NSW Premier's Literary Award and was listed in the American Library Association's 2010 Best Books for Young Adults. Its sequel, *The FitzOsbornes in Exile*, was shortlisted for the NSW and WA Premier's Literary Awards, named a Children's Book Council of Australia Notable Book and listed in *Kirkus Reviews'* Best Teen Books of 2011. The final book in the series, *The FitzOsbornes at War*, received starred reviews in *Kirkus Reviews*, *Booklist* and *The Bulletin of the Center for Children's Books* and was listed in *Kirkus Reviews'* Best Teen Books of 2012. Michelle has a science degree, worked as a speech pathologist for many years and is now a hospital administrator.

Visit www.michellecooper-writer.com for more information about Michelle and her books, including teaching resources.

www.ingramcontent.com/pod-product-compliance
Lightning Source LLC
Chambersburg PA
CBHW032026290426
44110CB00012B/684